THE DIARIES OF WILLIAM GATES

For Wadham College
January 2003

The Warden (Maurice Bowra)
said I was very distinguished, as
all the rest got through. It wasn't
for the want of trying!

William Gates

WILLIAM GATES

Born and educated in the county of Middlesex, the author went first to Fulwell Infants' School, then to Sunbury Council School and finally to Hampton Grammar School.

During the war, in the battleship HMS Malaya, he saw action against the Italian Fleet and later ran the gauntlet of German bombers and U boats while on Malta convoys.

Commissioned in 1942 he left the Navy at the end of the war and went up to Oxford where he read English Language and Literature.

After Oxford he went into his family business, Cow & Gate, then later worked for his younger brother, Alan, who owned employment agencies. Retiring at the age of 72 he began voluntary work at Westminster Childrens Hospital; when that closed he moved to Great Ormond Street Hospital for Children where he has been for the past five years.

In his 1953 diary, for January 6, he put: *I have written since I was four years old.* This need to write has been constant throughout his life, resulting in the Forsyth series, books based on the execution of a teenager in 1960. Three of these: **Violence, The Trial** and **501 Days** have been published; the fourth, **Vision of Glory**, is in preparation.

**This diary is dedicated to all the children
I have known throughout the years
in Great Ormond Street**

THE DIARIES OF WILLIAM GATES

Volume Ten

2000

DESTINATION WAY
2000

Published by
Destination Way
PO Box 7700
London, SW1V 3XQ
United Kingdom

Copyright © William Gates 2000

Second impression 2002

The right of William Gates to be identified
as the author of this work
has been asserted by him in accordance with
the Copyright, Designs and Patents Act 1988

All rights reserved. No part of this publication may be
reproduced, stored in a retrieval system, or transmitted, in any form
or by any means, without the prior permission
in writing of Destination Way, nor be otherwise circulated
in any form of binding or cover other than that in which
it is published and without a similar condition including this
condition being imposed on the subsequent purchaser

ISBN 0-9525896-3-X

Printed in Great Britain by

Bookcraft,
Midsomer Norton,
Bath

Contents

Contents

Preface

I have to admit that when I came into the world at 2.30 on the morning of 14 April 1919, adding one more human being to the 1,646,000,000 already here, I didn't know what I was in for. We all want to be someone, to be recognised, and only a few come in at the top. There must be people without a care in the world but I haven't met any, so for most of us the problem is simply staying alive.

Why people keep diaries I can't say. I can't say why I've kept these diaries. I've been pretty mixed up all my life and have failed almost everything I've gone in for, but I wouldn't want to swap my life with anyone else, nor would I want to live it again. If you have the sense to keep your personal diaries secret then no-one will see you as you really are. It's stupid, I suppose, to let people know you aren't the nice considerate person you hope they think you are.

People who really annoy me are those who become rich and famous and brag about their humble background. There's nothing to be said for being poor as any rich aristocrat will tell you. We were poor. My father separated from my mother, Freda, when I was three, returned to Ireland, to a comfortable life with servants and to his own idea of enjoyment, drinking and gambling. Because of this, because he was often short, he didn't send the £3 a week he was supposed to allow my mother for the four of us. But we were happy, Bobby, Jackie, John and I as were my half-sister and brothers, Babette, Alan and Ian who came along later. Jack was a wonderful step-father.

When I started reading through these diaries, having forgotten what I'd written, it came as a shock to find out what I really thought about everything. I was tempted to leave out the early obsession with death that so disturbed me, but realized that doing this was giving way to the old compulsion of wanting to show myself in a good light, to be what I'm not. During the war, at HMS *King Alfred*, when as cadets we were going through for our commissions, a senior officer told me that if he had his way he would get everyone drunk, watch their behaviour, then decide who would make an officer and a gentleman. Drink is a great leveller, so are diaries. In your diaries it's difficult to be the actor playing a role.

The past seems to stretch back interminably. Childhood, the Navy, University and fifty years of so-called peace; but when I look back one incident stands out above all the rest. It was a meal, a simple meal, but the best meal I've ever tasted. Claridges, the Savoy, the Ivy, Simpsons, all my old haunts, don't compare. It was after an action between us and the Italians and I have never forgotten the incredible feeling of relief when the bombs stopped whistling down and shells were no longer shrieking over, sending up huge spouts of water on either side of us; for the Italian fleet had retreated taking their dead and wounded back to base. I stood quite still on the bridge beside my rangefinder, cradled by the sudden quietness, the Mediterranean sun warm on my face, the terror of being at any moment blown to bits, over. I felt good. Then our young galley hand came up to where I was standing and, smilingly, handed me the tastiest wodge of corn beef sandwich ever and a large mug of delicious brown stewed tea.

It was good, it was really good, and it was just great to be alive.

2000

Tuesday January 4, Dolphin Square

I went to GOSH for Christmas Eve, Christmas Day and Boxing Day. For the New Year I went to John and Isobel (Doubleday). Robert, Edwin, James and their friends were there. I had a lovely time.

We lit a large bonfire in the grounds to see midnight in, and sent up a rocket half-a-minute before twelve - it burst right on time - and we gave three cheers. On my last day there, which was New Year's day, John and Isobel gave a lunch for twenty people and they opened a bottle of wine 150 years old. It had a sharp taste. Isobel's kitchen clock had packed up so, for her millennium present I bought a very nice clock from Peter Jones.

8.30pm. Have just returned from GOSH. Am too tired to write more now, but will do so tomorrow.

Wednesday January 5, Dolphin Square

Yesterday, Louise, aged 13, who was the victim of a road accident, came in and was put on a life-support machine in PICU. At 6.30pm, when I was on my ward rounds, I went into PICU and saw the family, about twenty of them, grouped outside her room. Two of them came over and told me she had just died. It was very sad. I don't know what the accident was; I can only assume she was knocked down.

In Alice Ward I went in to see James (W), aged 13, who will be 14 on 26 February. He had been sent to Frederick Still ward but returned to Alice. He has a rare illness, and is in constant pain with his lips and inside his mouth. The cause isn't known and different treatment is being tried. He is a delightful boy and told me that the constant pain is depressing him (naturally), and he can't sleep properly. He and his father have built an aviary, and he has got his first two birds. He had a paper all about birds, and I gave him £5 to get one. He was delighted and said he'd get a red canary which he would call William.

Samira (A), aged 6, in a wheelchair, was in GOSH with her mother. She is coming in on Thursday, to Parrot Ward, for her

11

fourteenth operation. She is a pretty little girl and has been through so much. I also saw little Lewis, in Helena, who today is going for his operation to have a Hickman line fitted, and for gastroscopy. Laura (C) is back on Clarence Ward. I'll see her again on Friday.

Yesterday morning I posted the opening chapters (revised version) of *The Vacuum Seal* to Gregory & Radice, which they asked me to do. If they reject them then that's that, and I will be disappointed but not surprised. I am used to rejections. If they ask to see the rest of the book then I will think I stand a reasonable - but not certain - chance of publication.

Thursday January 6, Dolphin Square

I had a pleasant day with Ali and Anita (Weinel). The children are lovely. I nursed Toby a lot. He is a beautiful baby. Eleanor is a bright child. Very attractive.

I had a card from Leon (Greenman), sent in 1999, but arrived this week. He thanked me for my voucher gift for his 89th birthday. He had written on a card which he designed himself, a drawing of him behind barbed wire in Auschwitz where he lost his wife and child in the gas chamber.

Friday January 7, Dolphin Square

Went into GOSH early and had lunch, as Andy and Jane are coming this evening. Christopher (S) is back again. I was very sorry to see him looking so poorly. He has leukaemia and went into remission. He's in Fox Ward so I can visit him there. It would have been difficult if he'd gone to Robin as most children in Robin are in isolation.

I also saw Emma (T). She was in Alice for the day. She has a bad skin complaint and is covered in white bandages. While I was there the Nurse had to insert a needle for a blood test; it was where Emma's ribs are and it hurt her, but she was OK once it was out. Her mother said that what she has, osteopetrosis, has made her bones soft and she's broken one in her foot and (I think) one in her arm. She's a beautiful girl, small for her age which is understandable as she's in a wheelchair all the time. She will be 15 in September.

Little Joe in Clarence Ward was very upset because he's had a frame put on his leg. I tried to comfort him by saying it was to make him better, but I don't think he was convinced.

I saw Samira in Parrot who had just returned from her fourteenth operation on her head. The Surgeon was William

Harkness. He was in the ward and we had a chat as he and I have been friends for many years - he said about twenty. He is a brilliant world-class neuro-surgeon. He got me into the operating theatre for a day where I saw him operate on a little four-year-old Greek girl who had a tumour on the brain, and a ten-year-old boy who had a leucotomy to stop him having fits. I will never forget my day there.

James (W) has gone home so I gave the M & S wine gums I had got for him to Emma; I'll get him some more on Wednesday and post them to him.

I bumped into little Zak (G) who was going to Elephant Day Care for a check-up. He had a bone marrow transplant some time ago. Laura has gone home from Clarence. I saw Tom there.

In Parrot was a teenage girl who had been knocked down by a van. She still seemed to be in a coma but I think was coming out of it. Her mother said she had head injuries - bruising of the brain.

This evening Andy and Jane took me to the local fish & chip shop for supper. We had a delicious meal and a very delightful evening.

I had a second card from Stephen (GOSH catering) from Australia where he is on holiday.

Saturday January 8, Dolphin Square

I've worked on my book *The Vacuum Seal* all day. I spoke to Rhoda (Milne). She has been taken ill, has been in great pain and couldn't move. I've had another order email for **The Trial**. It's now in quite a few of the leading law libraries, here and abroad.

Sunday January 9, Dolphin Square

I've been thinking about Christopher who has come back into GOSH. He looks so ill and I am very worried about him. He went through so much and for so long before he went into remission. I was thinking too of Emma and James. These poor children.

All day I've been working on *The Vacuum Seal*. Gregory & Radice may not want to go on with me, but if they do I would be prepared.

I spoke to June (Harkness) and told her what a wonderful son she has in William, who is a paediatric surgeon of world renown.

Sylvia (Gates) rang me this morning. John and Wendy had gone to a funeral in Wales. I also spoke to Rosie (Watts). She was fine. She is 89 in July and is wonderful.

Monday January 10, Dolphin Square

Bill (Richards) rang me for another sitting (for my portrait) which I am having on Wednesday. Bobby rang; he's been investigating the best soap for me to use, because of my skin, and we decided on Neutrogen.

Tuesday January 11, GOSH

Saw Christopher in Fox Ward. He is very tired but in the evening was a little better as he'd had an anti-sickness injection. I took him up a toy - a lovely and unusual one; with a beak and a smiling face. I told him it was his mascot and he could tell it all his troubles. I've done this before with very sick children and it is quite extraordinary how much it means to them, and the comfort it brings. On the label the name Percy had been written, so Percy he's been called. When I went up again later, Christopher had Percy on his pillow so I told him I would write to where Percy came from, Chessington World of Adventures, and let them know, which I now have done.

Emma (L), who works on reception for Robin and Fox wards, told me Ryan (P), who had leukaemia, has had a relapse and will be coming in.

In Dialysis I saw Mehmet (K) and got him smoky bacon crisps and whole nut chocolate. Freddie in Dialysis wanted a Kinder Surprise (a chocolate egg), and Matthew wanted Cheesy What's It (crisps). I also saw Riza.

AJ (McL) is back. He was in a wheelchair by the front desk and said he'd paged me.

In Victoria Ward I saw Florence (H), 13, who has had a kidney transplant. In Giraffe I saw Claire (H),10, who'd had a bone marrow transplant, and other children including Dean (H),13, and Kirsty (McD), 14, in DJW.

Thursday January 13, Dolphin Square

Yesterday evening I met Ali for a drink, near Earl's Court. His friend Brenton came then we went on to Chelsea. They didn't play very well but a new Nigerian striker, playing in his first Chelsea match, headed in a goal three minutes from the end.

If *A Light in the Yellow Hut* is not taken by Gregory & Radice who have the first two chapters, I'll send it to publishers for the slush pile. I'll also re-write it, still handwritten from 40 years ago.

Friday January 14, GOSH

I went into GOSH early, meaning to leave about tea-time but was asked to help Emma on the front desk; so I didn't get back until nearly 8.30pm and am tired. I will go on with this tomorrow.

To continue: I had a long day, but when I go into GOSH Tuesdays and Fridays, my time is theirs. I get plenty of time for my own work. Apart from GOSH I go out very little.

My main concern is Christopher. He is very ill, and it is worrying that the leukaemia has returned. I spent a lot of time with him and Vera, his Grandmother. While I was in his room a top Consultant came in. I think her name is Judith. She had two other doctors with her and I was allowed to stay. She told Christopher they were giving him treatment that would make him feel rough temporarily but will help eventually. I'll see Christopher again on Tuesday if I don't go in before.

Laura (C) is back in Clarence. She's had a pain in her leg (or hip) and they are investigating.

Pierre (H) had left a bottle of wine for me in my in-tray behind the front desk, and a card from Ann, Colin and Chantelle. I have written and thanked them.

Sunday January 16, Dolphin Square

I've still got a bit of a sore throat, but so far it's stayed like this. I'm now going to start copying out from the old MS, my novel *A Light in the Yellow Hut* and see if I can make something of it.

Monday January 17, Dolphin Square

I've had a super day. Went to lunch with Ingibjörg and Barry (Andrews). Inga works behind the front desk in GOSH. They have a lovely house in Hammersmith. Inga is very clever, she makes the most beautiful mosaic mirrors, animals etc.

I had a sore throat last night so gargled with TCP. Now I've got a head cold so am going to bed early.

Tuesday January 18, Dolphin Square

I felt so ill last night with the 'flu. I stayed in all day as I couldn't go to GOSH because of the children. I sent three Dolphin Square cards to Omar (A), Matthew (G) and Christopher (S). I feel a bit better but have sat most of the day in an armchair. Ayesha, Omar's Mum, sent me a lovely photo of him.

Wednesday January 19, Dolphin Square

I felt better today but still have a remnant of the cold. I got another order for **The Trial** from Durham University. I've heard no more from Gregory & Radice. Because of my cold I didn't go to French class this evening. Anne (Rivoire) my teacher rang me last night and I said I probably wouldn't go. I'm not going to GOSH this week.

Thursday January 20, Dolphin Square

I heard from Gregory & Radice. They turned down my book. Disappointing after they had said they were very interested. Also their letter, in contrast to the first friendly one, was cold. I'll get on with my diaries. I think I'll stop bothering with the commercial market. I've tried and tried and tried, and it wastes so much time.

Friday January 21, Dolphin Square

I am very worried about Christopher. Emma, who is on the front desk this evening, told me he is in PICU. Then I spoke to Vera, Christopher's Grandmother and she said he is on artificial breathing and has a catheter. He is asleep all the time. I haven't been in GOSH this week because of my cold; I hope to be back on Tuesday and will see him then.

I like Tony Blair, our Prime Minister. Not because he wrote me a personal letter, but because he has qualities I admire. He has had a bad time this year with NHS problems and rising crime, but he said he's not going to be deflected from what he's set out to do. I feel it's important to have this attitude. I've made up my mind to get out all my diaries, and also Book IV of the Forsyth series **Vision of Glory**.

Went to Moorfields this morning for my six-monthly check-up. My good eye has changed but it isn't serious; however, I'm going back in four months instead of six. I had a charming lady doctor from South Africa.

Saturday January 22, Dolphin Square

Had two more orders for **The Trial** from law libraries.
I spoke to Jane this evening to fix a Thursday for her and Andy to come to the Golf Club in February. We had quite a long talk and I said that with writing you can never tell what may happen. This evening there was a programme on Mervyn Peake. He was one of the greatest illustrators: I saw some originals in the Army

Museum, but his peculiar Gothic books didn't sell until after his death; now they are never out of print.

Had a card from Ann Huigbregtse, a successful American sculptor, who wrote:

How can I tell you how much I've enjoyed reading your diary, and then your Christmas letter comes and I've got a 1999 update. What fun! You are an inspiration.

This afternoon I rang PICU to see how Christopher is. The Sister said he's slightly improved.

Sunday January 23, Dolphin Square

I went over to see Sylvia, Wendy and John. Sylvia gave me tea and lamb sandwiches and we all sat talking in the front room. I enjoyed it very much.

During the war Bobby sent me, from Hong Kong, a Parker 51. I have used it for all my creative writing ever since, but now it's difficult to use as it goes in fits and starts. It has great sentimental value.

Monday January 24, Dolphin Square

I had such a nice letter from James (W) telling me about his aviary. Also one from Adam. We correspond regularly. I forgot to mention yesterday I spoke to Liz and James (P) on the telephone. James is coming into GOSH for a pelvis operation. He is 16 on 20 April.

Regarding Bobby's Parker 51, I'll go on with it unless it becomes too difficult.

Tuesday January 25, Dolphin Square

I saw Christopher in Intensive Care. He is very ill. Vera, his Grandmother, is with him all the time. I spoke to Scott, the male Nurse in charge of Christopher who is very nice. Mr Grove, of Grove International who manufacture beautiful toys, had written a lovely letter to Christopher and sent him Winnie-the-Pooh. I've written to Mr Grove to tell him the situation, and thank him.

Little Mitch is back in Fox. He is very bright and amusing.

Ben (C) had left me a note to say he was back in Alexandra Ward for his operation, so I went up to see him. I stayed until 8.00pm and saw quite a few children.

I had a long chat to Emma (L) who was behind the front desk. She supports Tottenham, I am Chelsea, and both teams are playing each other Saturday week.

I've been feeling a bit low these last few days. I watched the Whitbread literary awards last night, so many successful writers; but how about all the unsuccessful ones, and there are so many of these? I framed an insurance advert which says: **THE WILL TO WIN IS NOT ENOUGH, YOU NEED TO APPLY YOURSELF.**

Bill (Richards) finished my portrait today. It is excellent. He has started on the second. When I said to Bill other people's problems are, usually, worse than one's own he dismissed this and said it's your own problems you have to think about.

Today it was announced there will be a remembrance day for the Holocaust. Good.

Thursday January 27, Dolphin Square

I had a very pleasant visit to Grays in Essex for a luncheon given by the Rotary Club of Grays Thurrock, to receive a cheque from them for GOSH. Peter Brainwood was there and others I had met when I went before. I enjoyed it very much. I was shown the way there by a charming woman called Margaret who lived not far away, and who was walking in the direction I had to go. She told me about her son and two daughters and it was nice meeting her. She was carrying a large pink lampshade she had bought. I think one can get a lot out of casual meetings, and learn a lot.

When I got back from the Rotary Club there was a message on my answering machine to ring Salina (T). It was to tell me Anne Mackie had died about midnight. Anne was Supervisor at GOSH front desk when I started there. She was a lovely person, a beautiful nature always helping people, never a bad word about anyone. She had leukaemia.

10.30am. Am just going into GOSH. Hope Christopher is OK.

Friday January 28, Dolphin Square

Christopher has gone back to Robin Ward. I spent a long time with him. The Nurses were with him quite a lot. He was in constant pain, saying his tummy hurt and his back, and he couldn't hear. Vera, his Nan, I and the Nurses comforted him as much as we could. He did sleep at times, but he can only have so much morphine. He has various lines attached from his body to the machine by his bed.

When I arrived at GOSH in the early afternoon Millie, who was on duty at the front desk told me a child in PICU had died and I thought it was Christopher. I always feel awful hearing that any

child has died, but of course it makes it worse when you know the child as well as I know Christopher.
I saw Ben (C) in Alexandra.

Saturday January 29, Dolphin Square

Had a sitting with Bill for my next portrait, then I went to GOSH and saw Ben and Christopher. Ben wasn't too well and wanted to sleep. I gave him some nectarines. Christopher looked a little better but is still very ill. Vera was with him.

Sunday January 30, Dolphin Square

I often think of myself as a failure. Never passing exams, never getting anywhere in business. Yet so many of those who succeed seem to fade and become one of the great crowd who are unknown except among their own little circles. Most are happy being this way, with their families. I'm 81 in April. Hoping is the secret of living: always hoping.

Monday January 31, Dolphin Square

Bobby's Parker 51 sometimes writes very well and flows well, as it does now.
Last night I sat up and watched a film based on a true incident. An American patrol in Vietnam kidnapped, raped and murdered a local girl. One decent young recruit brought them to justice.
On the news was one of our biggest mass murderers, Dr. Shipman, who was found guilty of killing fifteen elderly women but actually murdered many others, at least 150, probably a lot more. A lot of scheduled programmes were cancelled and the major part of the evening, on all stations, given over to Dr. Harold Shipman.

Tuesday February 1, GOSH

It has been a sad day. Nina, Nurse in DJW Ward, told me Vanessa (G) has been given only three months to live. Her leukaemia has returned. I've known Vanessa, 15, a long time and seen her a lot in her long illness. She has been taken on holiday to Florida. I've heard that at the moment she's quite well.
Then I went to Recovery to see Christopher who had just come out of theatre. He was rather miserable. A special bed has been got for him which costs £100 a day - so I was told. He is a very sick child. Scott, his Nurse in PICU, said there isn't much hope for his future. I feel deeply sorry. You get a very close bond with children

who are ill and with whom you share so much for so long.

Ben (C) in Alexandra Ward was also poorly. He has trouble with his bowel movements and gets very clogged up. He is also on what he calls his 'wee bag' and doesn't like having it, but I said it's to help make him better. He's an only child and has been coming to GOSH since he was a baby.

I saw little Michael in Lion. He has been in for a very long time. I'm not sure what is wrong with him. Lion is a cancer ward. He is nearly 5, I think. I'll check on it next time.

Emma (L) has offered me a lift in her car to go to Anne Mackie's funeral on Friday. I discussed it with Salina who is in charge of the front desk; it's been agreed I will go there under my own steam, which is easier. I only want to go to the service as I'm meeting Sue Collins in GOSH at 4.00pm. She is coming in to see one of her pupils who is in for ear surgery.

Christopher's Grandmother, Vera, has been reading extracts from my diary to Wendy, one of the GOSH social workers; Wendy told me she was once *au pair* to Norry and Ruth McCurry's children. Norry is in my diaries.

I met a very nice family. The patient is Helen (P), aged 20, unusual for GOSH but they will keep children on if they have been here for many years and the treatment is on-going. Her parents were with her. Mum has become very religious but the others aren't. Mum said she has a book with a daily prayer and she feels God's presence all the time. I am all for it. I wish I had this faith. Bobby has it.

Wednesday February 2, Dolphin Square

Had a sitting with Bill. He is not very pleased with the portrait at the moment, but this happened with the last one which is brilliant. I like this one, too, the way it is coming on.

I've been feeling a bit low these last few weeks, starting with the rejection by the literary agent of *The Vacuum Seal*. I'm feeling much better now.

ITV have just finished the concluding part on how Peter Sutcliffe, the Yorkshire Ripper, was caught. I went to the first day of his trial in May 1981 as I was researching at the Old Bailey and Liz Hart, who was in charge of administration, took me into No. 1 Court. All the knives and hammers he used to kill his women victims were laid out and labelled and, before he was brought up into the dock, there was a curious atmosphere of anticipation, the place packed with the Press and extra officers.

When he came up I looked at him and couldn't see him as a monster who killed; he looked quite ordinary, just as Denis Nielsen did when I saw him at his trial. Another murder trial that Liz got me into was that of 14-year-old schoolboy called Wood. He looked angelic, but when he was found guilty he screamed and screamed, all the madness in him showing. Wood had murdered a fellow schoolboy and buried him in the local churchyard. Before the trial I was told it was important he was found guilty, because had he been released he would have killed again. As well as the boy he murdered and buried, he had tried to kill another boy.

Thursday February 3, GOSH

I don't normally go into GOSH on Thursday but Iris (R) rang me to say she was bringing Sean in. I met her in the Dental Department. Sean is 16 next Wednesday. He is in a wheelchair all the time. He always looks as if he's asleep, but I don't know how much he understands. Iris and Michael, who adopted Sean, said that on two occasions recently, they thought they had lost him. Michael himself isn't too well: he has leg sores etc.

James (W) is back in Alice. The second time I went up to see him he was surrounded by the Consultant and his team. He still has the pain in his mouth. I also saw Ben (C) who is a little better. He's had his 'wee bag' removed and this had pleased him, so I was told. He was asleep, so I only stayed a short time. Maureen, Alexandra Ward Sister, came in and we had a chat.

The child who worries me a lot is Christopher, in Robin Ward. I don't think he's going to make it. I wish I hadn't got to write this, I hope more than anything that I'm wrong, but I can only say again that I'm very worried.

I had an early lunch then Ingibjörg , who works behind the front desk, and I went to the Italian Hospital where she was on duty until 4.00pm, and we spoke about my books. She likes very much what I write now, but is critical of *The Vacuum Seal*. She said the philosophising part needs taking out. We agreed that if I tried to do too much I would get nothing done. Two major tasks are to get all my diaries out and to finish Volume IV of the Forsyth books. This is what I will concentrate on, giving the diaries priority.

Friday February 4, GOSH

Christopher's Dictation - 1
Robin Ward 5.15pm

I am on a special bed which has buttons you can press - a bit uncomfortable and a bit all right.

I have had tummy pains at night for a long time.

William gave me £5 before I went to King's College Hospital the next day. William will visit me there.

Nan is staying with me in King's College Hospital.

I am going to King's College Hospital for a liver transplant. I am hoping it all goes well. I am at the top of the list for the transplant.

I would like to add some of the nurses' names who have been looking after me.

These are:

Jin-Hua

Sian

Rachel 1 & 2

Kirsty

Maxine

My older brother Kevin, aged 12, visits me often. I always like seeing him because he cheers me up.

I like it when Aunty Kay visits me because she helps the nurses when they do things with me, and she cheers me up. I like Nan being with me all the time because she helps me if I need anything.

The doctors are very nice and I saw the head one from King's College Hospital.

Kevin is at Shenfield High School where they teach the boys and girls separately.

Kay has three children: Amy, George and Alex.

(Signed) Christopher Smith.

Saturday February 5, GOSH

I wrote in my notebook what Christopher dictated yesterday, as I promised him I would. For the time I was with him he was awake and quite coherent. I was with him about half-an-hour at 5.00pm and I went back at 7.00pm. After my first visit Wendy, the GOSH Social Worker, took me to the parents room and explained that Christopher will die within two days unless he has a liver transplant. He is going to theatre today and will be put in a state of sleep for the next two weeks; then he will be taken to King's

College Hospital and will be given top priority for the transplant. There had been a meeting between Christopher's team of Consultant, Doctors, Nurses and Wendy and the top Consultant from King's. It was decided this is Christopher's only chance.

When I gave Christopher the £5 he said he'd put W in each corner of the note to remind him of me. I don't hold out a lot of hope for him, I only wish I could; and it is very harrowing to see him like this. I've known him for so long.

In Alexandra I saw Ben (C). He is looking a lot better. I gave him £5 which he appreciated. But £5 is nothing compared to the happiness it gives, not just so much the money but the pleasure of an unexpected gift. I don't lead any sort of social life, and people think nothing of spending £1,000 going abroad.

I also saw Charlie who'd had an operation on her face to remove a large tumour. She was in Tiger Ward and about to go home.

Sunday February 6, Dolphin Square

I've been thinking a lot about Christopher. If all has gone according to plan, he should now be in King's College Hospital. I also think of Ben (C) in Alexandra although he is not nearly as ill as Christopher. I also thought of little Michael in Lion and others.

Most of today I've continued clearing up a lot of things.

Marie (Rosie's daughter) telephoned. She'd been reading my diary and was enjoying it.

I wrote to Mr Mackinley MP who feels as strongly as I do, that an unconditional pardon should be given to the so-called deserters, the shell-shocked young men, including teenagers, shot in the First World War.

Monday February 7, Dolphin Square

I met Bobby at Feltham and we got the bus to Sunbury Village. We spent a pleasant couple of hours with Sylvia. (John and Wendy are in Goa on holiday); then Bobby and I walked back to Sunbury Village and got the bus to Kingston. It was really great being with Bobby and travelling along memory lane.

I've thought a lot about Christopher. I hope he's all right.

Tuesday February 8, GOSH

I saw quite a few children I have known a long time, who come in for out-patients appointments. Liz and James (P) were in, with Liz's sister Jill. Jamie had a scan: he has little bone lumps all over him, a genetic disorder. He will be 16 in April. Jill told me that she and her husband are moving to Florida. Liz will miss them particularly as they lost their brother recently, who collapsed and died - not very old. Some families do suffer so much.

Wendy, Christopher's Social Worker, said he misses me, so I'm going over to see him at King's College Hospital on Friday morning.

Ben (C) in Alexandra, gave me a beautiful 'thank you' card which he made on the school computer.

I saw little Jack (B) in Victoria. He had a kidney transplant a few days ago. He was lying naked, the long scar down his tummy. He is only 4. Eleri (H) in the same ward, was in theatre having a kidney transplant. When I left with Ingibjörg at 8.00pm she was in Intensive Care.

When I was having supper in the canteen Stephen, the young Superintendent there, sat with me and had a long talk. He was feeling low and was thinking of leaving the room he has in GOSH and renting a furnished flat, which would be a big mistake. He is having a reaction from his holiday in Australia. Anyway I got him round to thinking sensibly.

Wednesday February 9, Dolphin Square

French class this evening with Anne (Rivoire). She's a good teacher. I gave Ruth Watkins a brand new Kenwood mixer I'd bought but never used. She has just become engaged.

Thursday February 10, Dolphin Square

I had a pleasant day. Lunch with Kai and Irene Chung, then Andy and Jane came for dinner at the golf club. When I got back I saw a programme on TV on the Hubble space probe. The universe began six hundred billion years ago. Compare this to the span of our lives, and we are nothing.

Friday February 11, King's College Hospital and GOSH

This morning I went to Denmark Hill and saw Christopher who is in King's College Hospital waiting for his liver transplant. He is wired up to a machine; has almost nothing on and is yellow because of liver failure. Vera was there, and later Pamela, his mother came in and sat with her hand on his arm. Steve, the Play Specialist came in and he was very good and made Christopher laugh. Liz, Christopher's Nurse, took his temperature and blood pressure, she was very caring. He is in a large, very nice room.

Later Vera took me down to see Jenny, a GOSH Nurse (Robin Ward) who is quite ill with growths on her kidney and liver (I think); she has her operation on Tuesday. She wanted drinking chocolate, which they don't sell at King's, so I'll get her some and take it over soon.

In GOSH I saw Ben (C), who is now eating properly and was very bright and really bubbly. It was great to see him so well. Abdul is back in Alexandra. Both boys have cystic fibrosis. Ben is 15 on 20 May.

Ryan (P), aged 2, in Fox Ward has a particularly vicious type of leukaemia called AML. Unfortunately he has relapsed. Even with a transplant he has only a twenty per cent chance of survival.

Little Mitch (R), about Ryan's age, has gone into remission and is going home. His parents Mark and Melanie, are with him all the time. Mark, a car sales manager, hasn't been working to be with Mitch. People generally don't realize the stress for parents who have a very sick child. The father often has to stop work, not just to visit the hospital but to look after the other children. The stress is very great with always the worry and fear that the disease, such as leukaemia, will return.

I saw more children, then ended up at the annual Staff Party. The canteen was transformed, very colourful. I spoke to Robert Creighton, the Chief Executive, and others. I had a little wine, supper, and left just after 8.00pm. I enjoyed it.

Saturday February 12, Dolphin Square

I watched the first half of Chelsea v Wimbledon and bought a programme for Ali and Ben. Chelsea won but I don't yet know what the score was. Then I went to Denmark Hill, saw Christopher and, briefly, Jenny to give her the milk chocolate drink she wanted. She had two visitors including a GOSH play specialist. Christopher was much brighter and had lost the yellowness he had the last time. But we can't fool ourselves, he is a very, very sick child. Vera was with him.

This evening I did my laundry and was looking at glittering pictures of aristocratic girls, Lady Veronica this, and Lady someone else, all wearing exquisite dresses and looking glamorous; but I've seen so many of them away from the glitz, divorced, children with drug problems, depressed, ageing. Life is never what it seems.

To get back to Christopher. He will be 11 on 25 June.

Sunday February 13, Dolphin Square

I had the most awful news today. I had a message to telephone John (Doubleday). I did so and Isobel told me that Edwin had been killed yesterday evening, while travelling on the underground. He was on his way home and at Liverpool Street he got caught in the doors, was taken into the tunnel and crushed against the tunnel wall. I had only just written a letter to Edwin in answer to his email saying he would like to visit GOSH. I had told him I would continue his allowance until December, and that he was very welcome to come to GOSH and bring friends and other young doctors if he wanted to. He was my Godson, a medical student, and about to qualify as a doctor.

Later I rang John, got James, and said if John and Isobel wanted me to go for identification, which we hope will be tomorrow, I will do so. They said they'd like me to. Bobby is saying prayers for Edwin and the family. It is now 10.00pm and I still find it hard to believe this has happened.

Monday February 14, Dolphin Square

John and Isobel didn't have to go and identify Edwin as he had his passport, and they were told it would be very distressing. John said Edwin (who fell on the line) was decapitated along the waist and his legs crushed. His face is all right. It looks as if it was partly his fault, but it doesn't lessen the awfulness of what has happened.

Vera telephoned from King's College Hospital to say Christopher is going back to GOSH tomorrow.

Tuesday February 15, GOSH

Christopher's Dictation - 2
Robin Ward 7.00pm
At King's College I got an autograph of Gabby Roslyn, the TV Presenter.
My brother Kevin, aged 12, came to see me. Nan looked after me all the time. I liked it best of all when my Mum visited me.
Because my liver is much better I have been able to come back to GOSH quickly. I was in King's College Hospital a week and two days.
I will be eleven on June 25th 2000.
When I was in King's College they gave me a bear with a blue jumper so I named him after William.
I spoke to Kevin on the telephone (at GOSH) to see if he is going

to his Nan's in Norfolk, but he said 'no' to me. Now that I'm back in GOSH I've got the same nurses including Jin-Hua who is looking after me today.

I had a letter from Brenda and Hugh (Walker-Munro):
We were so sorry to hear about the terrible accident and death of your Godson.
And a card from them:
Thinking of you. We are so sorry.
Also a lovely photo of Edwin taken with Hugh by me when in Scotland.

THE TIMES, TUESDAY, FEBRUARY 15, 2000

Doubleday - *Edwin John Gordon, son of John and Isobel, brother of Robert and James, died suddenly on 12th February 2000 aged 23 years. Funeral Service at St Peter's Church, Great Totham, Essex, Friday 15th February at 3.30pm. Donations, if desired to Medecin Sans Frontiers 0171 713 5600.*

Wednesday February 16, Dolphin Square

I am stopping my voice mail answering service which is very unsatisfactory. I had four messages on it including one from Freddie not long before she died, wishing me a good new year. A short one from Anthony and one from America. The last one from James (Doubleday) which said:
Hullo, Bill, it's James Doubleday. It's about 1.00 o'clock on Monday and I was just phoning to say that we're not going to see Edwin today, partly because they are happy with him being identified by the passport and ID that he happened to have on him, and also because he was very badly damaged when he was killed and there's not much to see. So that's the situation. Thank you very much for offering to come with Mummy and Daddy. The funeral will probably be on Friday, this Friday afternoon. Thanks very much and lots of love. Goodbye.
All the other messages were wiped out because of a fault with the machine. I would like to have heard Freddie's again but it wasn't to be.
This evening I'm going to GOSH to see Christopher as I'm not going on Friday.
Had a card from Faith (J) today, who had seen Edwin's obituary in *The Times*.
8.00pm. Just come back from GOSH and seeing Christopher who is much brighter.

Christopher's Dictation - 3
Robin Ward
6.00pm

William came to see me today as he can't come in on Friday. I shall miss him not coming in on Friday.

Now I am back at GOSH I am feeling much better. I got up but I could hardly walk so I sat in a chair. If I want to get up I need someone to help me. The same with the bath: I sat in a chair and Kay wheeled me round to the bathroom and sat me in the bath and Jin-Hua helped me. After the bath my legs were aching but they are all right now.

Edwin's tragic accident was front page headlines in tonight's *Evening Standard*:

Horror of Student's Death on the Tube.
by Dick Murray and Patrick Gowan

A 24-year-old medical student, the son of a renowned sculptor, has been killed in a horrific accident on the tube.

Edwin Doubleday is believed to have been thrown to his death after he mistakenly remained on a train temporarily being taken out of service at Liverpool Street station last Saturday. For some unexplained reason Mr Doubleday, who was within three months of qualifying as a doctor, remained on the train.

Investigators believe he realized what had happened, left his seat near the front of the train and began to rush through the carriages via the inter-connecting doors. At that stage the platform would probably still have been in sight. The train passed over track points, causing the carriages to sway and jolt violently at the precise second, it is believed, that Mr Doubleday opened the connecting door and trod on the steel joining plates - which then jack-knifed, throwing him on to the lines.

Older brother Robert, 25, said today that Edwin's clothing was seen to catch in an inter-connecting door of the Central Line Tube train as he tried to get off at Liverpool Street. He was pulled under the wheels and died instantly. Investigators had to examine two trains and a number of carriages before establishing whether the medical student had fallen or was "catapulted" to his death.

Edwin was within three months of qualifying as a doctor and died while travelling from Manchester to visit his family at Goat Lodge Farm, Great Totham, Essex. He was the son of sculptor John Doubleday whose statues include Sherlock Holmes in Baker Street and Charlie Chaplin in Leicester Square.

The second of three sons, Edwin attended the Anglo European School at Ingatestone. Headmaster Bob Reed paid tribute to someone whom he described as a brilliant student with a wicked sense of humour.

Edwin went on to St Andrew's University, Scotland, to begin his medical studies and then went on to complete his training at Manchester University. Many fellow students are expected to attend the funeral at St Peter's Church, Great Totham, tomorrow. It will be taken by the Vicar the Rev. Michael Hatchett, a friend of the family. Today it was alleged that London Underground did not carry out a physical check with staff walking through the carriages, as it is claimed should have been done, to ensure they were empty.

Instead the driver, who is not being blamed, obeyed LU instructions to announce three times over the loudspeaker system that all passengers must disembark.

Bobby Law, a senior official with the Rail Maritime and Transport Union, accused LU of flouting safety regulations in not making sure the train was empty before it left the station to turn round. Mr Law said: "That man should never have been left on the train. LU did not have a member of staff on the platform to check the carriages.

"This is despite a clear warning by the Health and Safety Executive that trains must be checked by platform or on-board staff," he added.

"The Union has said for years that LU must return staff to platforms and guards on trains but they refuse, on cost grounds. This is the result."

Stanley Hart, HSE principal inspector of railways, ruled in a letter dated 22 November to LU: "Some time ago, HMRI (Her Majesty's Railway Inspectorate) raised the issue of passengers being overcarried into sidings or depots.

"The LU response was that trains were checked when the train was being taken out of service and not necessarily when reversing via a siding. This is not acceptable."

An LU spokesman confirmed the carriages had not been inspected but denied safety rules had been broken.

Thursday February 17, Dolphin Square

I had a letter this morning from John James Chambers, President of the Liverpool Beatles Appreciation Society, asking if I would incorporate his letter in my diary. I have known him for many years, and have always admired his dedication and enthusiam. He has written to and had replies from many distinguished public figures, and has appeared several times in his local paper in support of the

29

Beatles. Writing in his own inimitable way, which I wouldn't want to alter, his letters not only give an interesting account of his activities, but paint a colourful picture of Livererpool life:

how is your handwriting, its still good i think, from your last letters.

this has been typed with one finger. ttfn . cheers .

ps

yours letters diary book, sounds like it will be very exciting, with your various letters from these people, from years gone by, pps, there is a old man by us, a Mr john campbell, aged now 90 Ninety years of age, he lives at the top of our rosd all hes life, he lives with hes ill wife & is her carer, he is only a little man with a walking stick, who is still very mobile, & who goes to the shops for shopping the newsagents for hes paper & the post office for hes pension, i think its Wonderfull. / Absolutely wonderfull to se these old folk, out and about, my poor old MUM helen now aged 88 cant walk now and is very incontinent, but her mind is still sound, compus mentis.

I am typing this letter on one of your old letters, i would still like som of them Dolphi square postcards of you, you can invice me for them if need be thankyou, also id still like to obtain a copy of your book 501 Days, where can i obtain a copy and what price is it also have you any news / yet of the write up that you was going to do on us the society L B A S 1977 - 2000 millenium & the fans / in your planned new book diary/letters. / i am enclosing for you an (SAE) hope your keeping well in health bill, whenever I mention your name to anyone, they think I mean the other bill gates from america, the pc, microsoft boss, / ps what is your latest book project now / also do you ever here from sculptor john doubleday, and what is he working on now, also could you get us off john, a new signed dated photograph, for our proposed planned still, LBAS years history book, words / pictures, i got a nice autographed photo of george martin sir george, of Beatles recording fame, abbey road studios / ive made a start on both books storys the Beatles fans L B A S story & my carers book story, the lone carer 365 days imagine, / on both Rough (Manuscripts,) but work has stopped on this due to lack of funding money £, as i had to pay the computer operator woman mrs Ross. ROZ / a londoner living here. now, £10 . . out of my dole money, that is my DHS / S S income support and my (CARERS) allowance for being a full time carer, to my mum, whose not been well of late, and ive had my own personal problems not a very good year so far, / hope my our luck cheanges soon, for the better in every way,

/ paying ROZ £10 .. for say three hours work, shes managed so far to type out rintout the storys, both Rough Drafts M A N U S C R I P T S / she's very good with words nd feels that i am Born writer & Creative writer / amateur novice writer, ps / Bill i know that i have this unbelievable (Imagination) for Dreaming up storys fact & fiction, / Fantasy and Reality, & that i could be a TV scriptwriter after seeing the kind of scripts storys that the , TV soaos dish up, one of Brooksides scriptwriters comes from norrisgreen where i live, sean duggan, / i still to need to fond say a Ghostwriter to put my storys into the correct context. / i dont have this edge, thi professionalism please respond to all the points in my letter thank you john.

Friday February 18, Dolphin Square

Ali has just telephoned to ask how I am. He is very upset over Edwin because, although he didn't know him, he knows John and Isobel. John did a bronze bust of him when he was about 8; I took him to Wivenhoe for sittings. Derek and Pamela Collins sent condolences. I am catching the 12.47 to Witham.

9.30pm.I've returned from the funeral. There were well over 300 people. It was very harrowing. John and Isobel were in tears a lot. Robert and James very near it most of the time. Edwin is a terrible loss. He will leave a big gap in my life. He will always be with me. It was terrible seeing his coffin lowered into the grave. Edwin's family will never be the same. It has not completely destroyed them, they are too sensible to let that happen, but it has destroyed the family as it was. Edwin was such a lovely person in every way. Yet even if he had not been, to lose a son is terrible. I was talking to George and William, Andrew Doubleday's children; they had lost Tom the middle brother (as Edwin was) who died of drugs, and he is missed greatly.

There is a big article about Edwin in the *Telegraph*, also one in the *Mail*. And it has been a subject on the radio.

Saturday February 19, Dolphin Square

Bobby came today and fixed up my new answering machine. On the way he'd had a fall, tripped over the edge of the pavement so he went back and had an early night. He said he was OK but I'm a bit worried about him. He's not far off 80.

I've had quite a few telephone calls about Edwin. Isobel rang also. But I still feel a bit stunned. Betty rang too and Barbara Doyle-Davidson.

Sunday February 20, Dolphin Square

Went to Chelsea today for the first half of the match, mainly to get programmes for Ben and Ali.
I still can't get Edwin out of my mind. I never will. Rang Bobby. He said he's feeling better from his fall.

Monday February 21, Dolphin Square

Letter in tonight's *Evening Standard*:
Safety alert on train sleepers
THE official LU instructions to announce three times that passengers must disembark (Horror of student's death on the Tube, 17 February) are clearly inadequate. With one good reason - sleep.

How many times have we witnessed some travel-weary commuter, fast asleep at the end of a hard day's work?

The usual attitude when one witnesses such an individual is to play mental guessing games as to how far past their stop they may have gone.

Waking them up would go against tube etiquette. I know of at least one colleague who has ended up in the sidings as a result of some badly timed slumber.

Clearly an on-board check by staff should always be made.

If this were the case, then the recent untimely death of Edwin Doubleday on the Central Line could have been avoided.
Andy T Mahady
Shilling Place W7

Tuesday February 22, Dolphin Square

I saw Christopher but he was asleep. Vera said he's been sleeping a lot. I didn't stay long at GOSH as I went to a lecture in the British Library, hosted by Tim Day whom I hadn't seen for years. He is a very charming person who is responsible for the collection of tapes, including those of children (Andrew and Alastair), that I gave to the B.L. Sound Archive.

Wednesday February 23, Dolphin Square

I went to King's College Hospital and took Jenny, the nurse from Robin Ward, GOSH, some drinking chocolate. She's had a major operation. I got back to Victoria at 6.22pm so decided to go to the French class. I'm glad I did, I enjoyed it sitting between Ruth and Rachel, two lovely young girls. It took my mind away from dwelling on Edwin, which it has been all the time.

Thursday February 24, Dolphin Square

I gave a talk on GOSH to the Windmill Probus Ladies Luncheon Club. There were 75 ladies. It went well. One lady told me that her niece had been in GOSH with meningitis but sadly died at 21. The lady on my left said her grandson, a small boy, is autistic and mentally backward, and nothing can be done. He had also been to GOSH. It is such a mistake to think everyone else is problem-free. It's the opposite. Frank Jackson once said that if I went into a room with ten other people, I would be glad to come out with my own troubles.

Friday February 25, GOSH

I think Christopher is fading. I just feel he isn't going to survive. He sleeps a lot, opens his eyes now and then, and is just able to speak. I bent over him and he asked when I was going to see him again. I said Tuesday, but what I had told his Nan was that any time he wanted to see me I would go. He has a yellow look, his skin and in his eyes. No-one will tell you the truth about him; they can't, except his Consultant. I hope I'm wrong, but I don't think he'll go on a lot longer.

I saw Jack (P) in Lion Ward. He is 10 and a Wilms Tumour has come back on his lungs. He was just going down for his operation, which was postponed from yesterday as the special machine needed for the operation was being used for another of our little patients.

I also bumped into Pierre (H), who ran up, hugged and kissed me. He was looking well and I bought him some sweets. Ann, his mother, was with him. I can't remember exactly Pierre's age, it must be about 7.

Salina, who is in charge of the front desk, is leaving. She has got a management job at the Royal Marsden Hospital. I'm very fond of her and I'll miss her but she's done the right thing. GOSH is doing away with her job and, it seems, would have offered her a job in the telephone exchange. She's much too good for that. I think the front desk is going to alter completely with porters there. I'm glad I no longer work there. I enjoyed it while I did, but I wouldn't now.

Edwin is still very much in my thoughts. He always will be. Nettie Rolnick rang to say she's been thinking about him.

Getting back to Christopher, his mother, Pamela, was with him, which I was pleased about.

Saturday February 26, Dolphin Square

I still find it hard to believe what happened to Edwin. It seems unreal.

I'm getting on with my writing. There is so much to do, principally my diaries.

Sunday February 27, Dolphin Square

I rang GOSH and spoke to Kate, Staff Nurse in Robin. She said there's no change in Christopher , who was sleeping.

I'm getting fed up, or rather have got fed up with the swimming pool which has become noisy and crowded. In future I'll go to the gym and to the pool afterwards, then if it's too crowded I won't go in.

Isobel rang me this morning. They are being very brave over Edwin. She said Robert has won a Fulbright scholarship for a year in America if the university there will take him, and James has been offered a marketing job by Boots in Nottingham but he really wants to work in London. This evening I spoke to June Harkness and Betty Edwards who have both been very supportive over Edwin. I also spoke to Nettie. I spoke to Ali too, who has a sore throat and cold.

I want to concentrate on getting my diaries out. The idea came to me also to get out a book of children's letters (GOSH).

Monday February 28, Dolphin Square

I've been wondering today about Vanessa. She is 17, her leukaemia has returned and Nina, Staff Nurse in DJW Ward, told me Vanessa has been given three months to live and that she, as well as her family, knows this. I was with Vanessa all through her long treatment in GOSH. Nina said the family had taken Vanessa to Florida and she thinks I should write to them; but I feel if they'd wanted me to know they would have told me. It's terrible for them. I'll make some enquiries in Robin Ward tomorrow.

My proofs came in from Redwood today for Volume Three of my diaries. I showed them to Bill, when I went for a sitting; he glanced at them and said they look good. I think so, too.

Tuesday February 29, GOSH

12.45pm. Just had a call from Jane, Staff Nurse Robin Ward, to say Christopher is unconscious and the family want to see me. So I'll go straight in.

8.30pm. Christopher could go tonight. I spent some time with him - I went in three times. The first time his mother, Pamela, was with him, then Vera and Kay, also his brother Kevin. A Staff Nurse said they weren't expecting him to last out tomorrow. His body has taken so much and is simply packing up. He is a lovely child, only ten years old. I'll go in again tomorrow morning.

Wednesday March 1, Dolphin Square

A.J., Alexandra Ward, is a little monkey. He tried to sell me a camera for £5 which he said he'd paid a £1 for. I found out later from Peter, who has run Radio GOSH for over twenty years, that the camera was given to A.J. as a prize. Peter said that A.J., who has cystic fibrosis (which I knew) is on oxygen continually and is on borrowed time. It's now 7.00am and I'm going into Marks early, as I'll go into GOSH again today to see Christopher.

2.30pm. I've been with Christopher. He is in a coma. If his support were taken off, he wouldn't live. He is nearing the end. I was with Vera and Kay for a time, then with Pamela, his mother. It is very sad. He is peaceful and his breathing, although jerky, is easy. Pam, one of the Staff Nurses, is looking after him during the day. I read to Pamela Christopher's dictations. She was very moved. I said I'd type them out over the weekend and send them to her. She just stood holding Christopher's hand.

Thursday March 2, GOSH

I saw Christopher this evening. He has gone down hill, is in a coma with an oxygen mask although Sue, one of the nurses, said the mask doesn't do much. I held his hand but of course there was no response. He is nearing the end, and although it will be traumatic for the family when it happens, it's not as bad as this waiting for the end to come. Kerrie, another of Christopher's nurses, was in the room with him. Vera and Kay came in. Last night he had been very poorly and I gather they thought it was the end, and had telephoned a lot of people.

I also saw little Ryan whose leukaemia treatment has failed and there's not much hope for him.

Friday March 3, Dolphin Square

Christopher has taken up a lot of my time this week and rightly so. He has priority over everything else. This morning (it's now mid-day) I've been working on the proof of Volume Three of my diaries. I am going to have a bread-and-cheese lunch and then go into GOSH. I've worked out a better and easier system for visiting the wards.

I got back here at about 8.45pm. There was a delay on the Victoria line as a woman had fallen under the train at Pimlico. The person in the ticket office there told me he thinks she was alive. She had been smoking and refused to put out the cigarette when told to do so.

I saw Christopher twice. I held his hand and noticed it was no longer warm. Not exactly cold but hardly warm. Sabrina, another of his nurses, explained to Vera, Kay and me that when the body deteriorates the blood goes to the most important parts such as the brain. Christopher has to have his oxygen mask on now. He is in a coma, lying propped up on his pillow, breathing jerkily. I cannot see how he can last much longer. Vera said they hadn't expected him to last this long.

I am due in GOSH again on Tuesday but will go Monday, as Ben left a message on my answering machine to say he'd be in then. I told Vera to telephone me any time if they want me to come in.

Saturday March 4, Dolphin Square

6.30pm. Have just rung Robin Ward and spoke to Mary, a Staff Nurse. She said Christopher is deteriorating and had been taken off antibiotics. I've left a message for the family to say if they want me to go in tomorrow to let me know. But I may go in anyway. I don't think Christopher will go on for much longer.

Sunday March 5, Dolphin Square

With my writing, I am quite happy about that. I am going to concentrate on getting out all my diaries, which is a big job. It's now 10.30am and I'm going into GOSH to see Christopher.

2.45pm. I got back here from GOSH half-an-hour ago. When I got there I met Kay who had left a message on my answering machine, which I just missed. She told me Christopher died about 11.30 last night, and they sat talking to him so that he wouldn't feel alone. Vera was there and Wendy, the Social Worker. Pamela came in but I didn't see her.

I saw Christopher in the mortuary. Sue, a Staff Nurse, let me in. It's the first time I've been in there. He was tucked up in bed in a corner of the room. The stairs were carpeted and it didn't have the feel of a mortuary - simply but nicely furnished. He looked very peaceful, his eyes closed, his mouth just a little open. On his upper lip were fine hairs due to the drug tablets. I kissed him on the forehead, which was cold. They want me to go to the funeral. I don't like funerals but I will go to this if it helps the family.

I loved Christopher, as I love all the very sick children I deal with. It is a special kind of love, not one to be explained but I know it means a lot to them just as it does to me. The message on the answering machine, which I put on when I got back said: *Hello William. Just phoning to tell you that we lost Christopher last night. I'll keep hold of your number and I'll give you a ring tomorrow evening. Christopher is in the Chapel of Rest at Great Ormond Street and if you did want to see him obviously you are welcome to see him, otherwise I'll give you a call tomorrow evening.*

5.15pm. Margaret has just rung, then Bobby. Today is the anniversary of Ma's death. I hadn't realized it, but I'll never forget her, ever.

7.00pm. Bobby has just rung again. He said Ma died nine years ago.

Monday March 6, Dolphin Square

I'm having a clean-out. It's quite a slow process but is badly needed. I came across a letter, written years ago (it has 10th August but no year) from Mrs Walker-Munro. I had written and asked her if she could tell me about Rhinefield in the New Forest, where the Walker-Munros lived when I first met them. Her writing isn't all that easy to read but I'll do my best to relate it. It was written from Drumfork, the Walker-Munros Scottish home near Blairgowrie:

I will tell you all I know about Rhinefield.

The architect was Romaine Walker - he also built a rather ornate house in Park Lane, still there, Bucklands Manor. It joins Spanish Place. His planning I thought, and all his detail superb. My Mother-in-law didn't like antiques or oil pictures. She had some from the family but wasn't interested. Her carpets and china couldn't be bettered - she was very house proud. There must have been about 13 servants not counting electricians, carpenter, chauffeurs and fourteen gardeners.

To start with, when my in-laws first married they entertained tremendously, but my father-in-law (Lionel Walker-Munro) was a sick man. They built the house at the sea and used to take parties over, but more and more went there for the summer.

Again when I first remembered Rhinefield it was beautifully done, everything perfect but rather dead; the house only became alive when we all went there, fewer servants but much more cheerful. The hot house atmosphere went when my in-laws died.

> *That is really about all I can tell you about Rhinefield.*
> *Pat and Mary are here. Mary is making progress.*
> *With my love - Morna*

On 24 August 1978 (it was August 1978 when Mrs Walker-Munro wrote) I had a letter from Hampshire record office, which included this:

The house you mention seems also to have been known as Rhinefield Lodge. This house lay some two miles to the north-west of Brockenhurst and is the only one in the area to include Rhinefield in its name.White's County Directory of 1859 shows John E. Nelson, forest nurseryman, as the occupier and it was still a nursery in 1872.

3.30pm. Not long ago I telephoned the Coroner, Mr Barry Tuckfield. He knew immediately about Edwin and said it was a chance in millions it should have happened. He was very kind, said the inquest wouldn't be for at least a couple of months, that it would be public with a Jury and I have to telephone in about six weeks to see if they have a date. I want to go to it. He said they have released the body, as identification wasn't needed, and it would have been distressing to see Edwin.

This evening I went to GOSH to see Ben.

Tuesday March 7, GOSH

I don't suffer from black depressions but lately I've felt how useless and pointless, in the long run, life is. Why should Christopher have to die at the age of ten? The family were in again and Kevin, his 12-year-old brother, went to see Christopher in the mortuary. It was Kevin's choice and it was right to give him that choice.

Wednesday March 8, GOSH

I saw Ben yesterday in GOSH. Also A.J. I bumped into Ben as he was going home, wearing his Chelsea strip. He gave me a hug. A.J. does this too although both are (I think) thirteen. But a Nurse in Robin said the children are very fond of me. I am fond of them, which explains it. I saw quite a lot of children including Stephen (Q), aged 16, in Alice Ward, who has EB, a major skin problem. His arms are completely bandaged. He is from Co. Donegal. Today I got some chocolate caramels from Marks which I'll post to him as he's going home. In Fox Ward Immanuel (P), aged 2, is having tests for suspected leukaemia. I saw Ryan, too, who may not recover as he's not fit enough to have a bone-marrow transplant. Good news on baby Natasha who is getting to the end of her treatment for leukaemia; she and her Mum have been in GOSH for six months. It's a long hard treatment. Craig (B) was in Elephant Day Care. I dealt with him a lot when he was having his treatment for leukaemia. He was in for a check-up and looked well. Alenka (R) was in Victoria Ward with a kidney disease. In Parrot Ward I saw David (F), 11+, son of a Jewish couple who are very charming; he'd been operated on for a brain tumour.

I finished correcting the printed proof of Volume Three of my diaries and have sent it back to Peter.

Thursday March 9, Dolphin Square

I have been working on the disc (putting in Rhoda's corrections) for Volume Four of my diaries. I am so fortunate to have Rhoda. I don't know what I would have done without her help.

Friday March 10, GOSH

Met John, Helen, Hannah and Andrew (B) at 2.00pm. They had telephoned me here to say they were coming in. Before I went to GOSH, Kay (Christopher's Aunt) telephoned to tell me about the funeral arrangements for next Friday. She asked if Kevin, Christopher's 12-year-old brother, could write to me. Of course he can. I get lots of letters and cards from GOSH children.

In GOSH I saw little James (D), aged 6, in Alice Ward. He has EB (Epidermolysis Bullosa). In Alexandra Dominic (K) is back for his period check-up. He is 12 or possibly 13. I'll have to check his birthday. I gave him some chocolate buttons. He said he is a 'button boy'. Richard (O), 17, is also back for his check-up. He was very depressed and wanted to go to Jersey where his father lives. He thinks he is only in for three or four days, but Maureen (Alex Sister) says he's in for two weeks, which is needed for the check-up. Abdul and A.J. have gone home. George (F), nearly 6, is also in Alex but not for long. David (H) was still in Louise Ward. I gave him some more wine gums. He had made me a lovely 'thank you' card. He is nearly 11. Margaret, his mother, told me he'd had cancer of the bladder, so they took all this away and made him a new bladder out of his intestines. He is going home tomorrow. Stephen (G) had gone home from Louise so I posted his 'rocks' (sweets from Marks) and posted chocs to the other Stephen (Q), who was in Alice.

In Fox baby Natasha's Mum Claire took photos of me with Natasha on my lap. She is now about eight or nine months. She was five months when she came in, but the course lasts for six months with lots of ups and downs. But at least there is this chemo treatment now. In Victoria I saw Jimmy (W) and gave him the 'rocks' he wanted. I saw also Ashley (R), 15; and gave him money to get sweets. Sarah (R), 14 I think, who had a blood disorder had gone home.

In Helena I saw little Mara (G) who was happily squatting on the floor tearing up a magazine which she loves doing. Fay, her Grandmother, told me what is wrong with her; but there are so many things I can't remember them. I'll ask again. She (Mara) has been in GOSH, all but a few weeks, for (I think) a year.

At the front desk I saw Rita and Millie. I think there are going to be a lot of organisational changes in May.

Saturday March 11, Dolphin Square

This evening I watched on TV the story of Station X; the history of those brilliant people who broke the German code in World War Two and saved thousands, probably millions, of lives. One sad thing is the most brilliant of them committed suicide in (I think) 1954 because he was homosexual and was being persecuted. Terrible. But the programme took me right back to the war years, to the D Day landings when, from the Isle of Wight Combined Ops base at Yarmouth, I heard the aircraft that night roaring overhead on their way to France for D Day. Actually it's been an evening of war nostalgia with Dad's Army shown at 5.30pm; Station X at 7.00pm, and now the Beethoven Emperor Concerto is being played on the radio, which also takes me back to those days when I was attached for a short time to the officers' mess in the Army Barracks at Rainham, Kent, and where I was nearly kicked out of the mess for playing (on records) almost non-stop, the concerto; and at Rhinefield where, when I was by myself, I played it again and again on the old-fashioned radiogram in the little ante-room off the main hall.

Jackie's birthday.

Sunday March 12, Dolphin Square

11.30am. Have just had a long talk to Rosie who will be 89 next birthday (July). She loves talking about the old days and has been telling me about my childhood, when we had a very large house, The Bays, at Hampton Wick in Church Grove opposite Bushey Park. Bobby and I used to walk through the park to Hampton Grammar School.

Rosie said Mother used to let the rooms to actors and actresses from the Kingston Empire. The Bays and the Kingston Empire have been pulled down and built over. The Empire was near Kingston Station.

Ma's lodgers who came regularly were Gracie West (small in build) and Ethel Revrell (tall and lanky), and they acted as a pair at the Empire. Also Stanley Black who was then a young pianist but became a famous dance band leader.

But what was most interesting, she remembered Stephen Ward. She said he was a very quiet, softly spoken person. He was very good at drawing caricatures, which he did at the Empire. Rosie said (when much later the Hever Castle affair blew up) he was made a scapegoat, but I am sure he was murdered. She said he had a small room on the second floor down. Later, the papers said he had drawn brilliant caricatures of the Royal Family.

Rosie said there was also a Russian Prince who was a lodger; he was a trainee chef at The Mitre restaurant, Hampton Court. There was also a Chinaman who was spotlessly clean and had the most beautiful Chinese girl friend.

The rooms mostly were large. One had a billiard table. There was also what was then called the scullery with a big cooker and a long narrow sink.

Mother did the cooking and Rosie did the work from top to bottom once a week. There wasn't a lot of furniture, the rooms just had a bed, cupboard and chest-of-drawers. Steps led down from the middle floor to the garden which was large at the back, very small in front.

There were three boys on the top floor. Stephen Ward's room was on the floor underneath. There were quite a few women actresses who stayed from a week to three weeks. Rosie said when the lettings started we children slept in the basement. The food was very ordinary but Rosie said that's probably why we are all so healthy. One day she had to cook our meal and all she could find were sausages, so we had sausage and mash. I remember the day we got to The Bays and we all had thick slices of bread-and-butter and jam. But we were happy and had a good childhood. Rosie said that there were two Belgian boys - refugees, and a French girl, Georgina. She (Rosie) certainly has a marvellous memory. She said that when she was 16 she came to Winchendon Road and baby-sat for Ma.

Monday March 13, Dolphin Square

It's 11.00am and I'm just getting ready to go to Marie who wants to interview me, in connection with her studies.

Tuesday March 14, GOSH

Met William Harkness this evening who said he was very sorry to have learnt about Edwin. June (his mother) must have told him. Ben is back. He's been put in Alice Ward as Alexandra has a bug. He doesn't look well. I'll find out more on Friday. Adam (F) is also back in Clarence. He is 14 in July and is having an operation on his foot tomorrow. I saw Richard (O) in Alexandra. He is still looking depressed. He is 17 which could be the reason he is unhappy - no patients of his age for company.

Wednesday March 15, Dolphin Square

Had two sittings for my portrait with Bill. He did the eyes this morning and said they're the best he's ever done.

Thursday March 16, GOSH

Emma was on the front desk. She is 22 and very pretty.
I saw James (P) who is having a major operation tomorrow; also Adam (F) who had his operation on his foot. I met Steven (C), 12+, very nice-looking who has a growth problem. Jake (S) is back in Parrot to have his shunt renewed. His family, including his little brother Jos, were with him. I also saw in Parrot Sinead (L) aged 9. She has a recurrent brain tumour which affected her speaking.

Friday March 17, Dolphin Square

Today we said goodbye to Christopher. Among the many mourners were nurses and other staff from Great Ormond Street. Carrying it lightly on their shoulders, two of the undertakers brought the small white coffin into the church. After the service groups of people stood in the sunshine as the coffin was lowered into the grave. There were many flowers including a large wreath from Christopher's school; three teddy bears made from yellow petals laid out at intervals; also, made from white and blue petals, a match-size football.

Sunday March 19, Dolphin Square

This evening I watched a TV programme on Proust. Every day I read a little of him. There were some interesting comments from Alain de Botton and Louis de Bernieres, who wrote a brilliant novel called *Captain Corelli's Mandolin*. Some of them were:
1   *We don't learn anything until we are in pain or there is a problem.*

2 *A little insomnia is not without its value in making us appreciate sleep.*
3 *We only become positively inquisitive when we are distressed.*
4 *Friendship is a lie. It leads us to believe that we are not immediately alone.*
5 *What we really think is what we really are.*
6 *Taking conversation for reality is a waste of time.*
7 *It is irrelevant whether others are intelligent as long as they are kind.*
8 *The way we speak is linked to the way we feel.*
9 *Our dissatisfaction could be because we fail to look properly at our lives.*
10 *Deprivation drives us into a process of appreciation.*
11 *The onset of jealousy is the only thing that can rescue a relationship ruined by habit.*
12 *Books can be quite dangerous for you. If we use them for our guide we will miss out a lot of things going on in our life. We would like the author to provide us with answers when he can only provide desires.*

Tuesday March 21, GOSH

I saw all my usual young friends in Alexandra - Dominic, Nathan and A.J., also more, whom I've known a long time, in Dickens: Freddie, who was being filmed for a TV programme; Riza, Michael and Colette. All have to go on the dialysis machine three times a week.

On the way into the hospital William (Harkness) caught up with me and we walked along together. He is an old friend - I knew him when he was a medical student. He is now one of the world's leading neuro-surgeons. He got me permission to be with him in the operating theatre for two brain operations, in the morning a four-year-old Greek girl who had a large tumour, and in the afternoon for a leucotomy on a ten-year-old boy to stop him having fits.

Wednesday March 22, Dolphin Square

Although we have very sick children at GOSH, and the parents particularly are under great stress, you do see the very best of life. A child is a child regardless of race and religion. All that matters is to do everything possible to make the child better. I couldn't help reflecting on this when I read about a distinguished Austrian medical professor, Gross, who, during the war, wore

Nazi uniform with jackboots, and who killed mentally-handicapped children. The chief doctor of the clinic was hanged for his war crimes in 1946. Gross, who assisted him, escaped punishment because his own crimes have just come to light. The trouble is that he is 84 and doddery. I hope he can be brought to trial and, if found guilty, hanged. It is said he killed 72 children out of a total of 772 murdered for brain experiments etc. Awful.

Friday March 24, GOSH

Went to Salina's farewell party in the boardroom. It was a super party and I enjoyed every minute of it. Salina was Supervisor behind the front desk when I worked there. She is only 22, very attractive, and a lovely person to work for. I will miss her.
The father of a sick child told me the hospital is a sad place. I disagree with him. It is sad that children are ill. It's a happy place where the children, unless incapacitated, laugh and play. But to be fair to him his remarks were probably triggered by Andrea, aged 3, who was lying on a blanket on the floor. She has muscular dystrophy, she can just about move, doesn't speak and will only open her eyes if spoken to in a direct manner. Her mother said she is lucky to have lived so long.

Sunday March 26, Dolphin Square

The hour has gone on so we've got the light evenings. Sylvia rang and said they were doing a lot in the garden now. A Birmingham tragedy. Three teenagers burnt to death in a garden shed, which they'd made into a den for the night. They had used candles, which set fire to the bedding and they couldn't get out because there was no handle on the door. The uncle of one of them, Matthew Collins, said they were deeply shocked.
Wrote to little Emma (H), a GOSH patient. I get quite a few letters from children and always write back.
Had an hour's swim this morning. Very quiet in the pool and I enjoyed it.

Monday March 27, Dolphin Square

Mr Putin has become the new President of Russia. He looks as if he can put the country right - the crime and corruption - which badly needs doing.
Here there are the amusing activities of those competing for Mayor of London. It wouldn't surprise me to see Ken Livingstone get it. He was interviewed on TV yesterday and his answers to pointed and tricky questions would be unequalled anywhere.

Tuesday March 28, Dolphin Square

There was a message on my answering machine from Sylvia. I have never before heard her speak as she did this time, and for so long. I had sent her Christopher's dictations, and the design for the back cover of Diary Volume Ten, which has his photo on it. Her message was:

It's Sylvia, I got the letter about Christopher this morning, thank you very much, and I think it's very good, and I think that his Mum and family will be very proud that it's being kept alive in Diary 2000. People are so - you know I'm going back to when John died, I just didn't want him to be forgotten and I don't think Christopher will be forgotten in your book.

Then I got this card from Faith Johnson:

Thank you for your letter. Christopher's dictations are some of the sweetest, saddest, bravest things I have ever read. I can see how fond he was of you and knowing <u>why</u> you couldn't visit him on Friday makes it all so much worse. It's lovely the way he includes everyone who looked after him.

I think the reason I couldn't see Christopher on the Friday was that this particular Friday was the day of Edwin's funeral. Of course I didn't tell Christopher the reason. Just checked in my notebook, and it was the reason. Edwin's funeral was Friday 18 February.

I went to GOSH today and saw James (W) with his Mum. He said he was feeling better and had a biopsy test but hadn't got the result. He said he'll keep in touch.

In Victoria Ward I saw Peter (C), aged 3, who has had kidney failure. Also Jimmy (W) who was looking bright and may go home on Friday and Alya (M), 14. She is very nice and I've known her a long time. She's just come back into Victoria Ward.

In Alexandra I saw Nathan (B-W). He was dashing all over the place, as usual. Very lively. Dominic has gone home. It's his 14th birthday Saturday. A.J. wasn't looking all that bright. I gave him the £1 I allow him each week while he's in GOSH. He was on his ventilator mask all the time, or a lot of the time, but this, I think, is for monitoring. In Dickens Ward I got Freddie and Riza a chocolate called Kinder Surprise, and I got Aysha chocolate buttons.

In Clarence I saw Halima (K), aged 15. She is having spinal surgery. She has cerebral palsy, no speech, and her back cannot stay upright without support. In Helena I saw Michael (W) who was looking better, also Mara who was with Fay, her

Grandmother. There was also the sweetest little baby, four months old, called William.

Steven, Catering Supervisor, sat with me when I had my dinner in the Peter Pan cafe. He always does if he's there. He's very nice and we get on well together.

Wednesday March 29, Dolphin Square

Today in Marks & Spencer (Pantheon) Kathy, who works in foods, said there was an account in the *Daily Mail* of a boy in GOSH who had been left, and he bled to death. I couldn't believe it, so I bought the *Mail* and found the article which took up a whole page. It doesn't look good, and spoke of a catalogue of errors, but we'll have to wait until May for the result of the enquiry.

The article said Matthew Sorrel, aged 8, was left on a trolley in the recovery room, crying in pain, and bleeding internally while doctors searched in vain for blood products which could have saved his life. He'd had a history of illness with his kidney, so I don't know what the report will reveal. It is terrible Matthew died, but I hope GOSH is in the clear. I know we carry out operations all day and every day, but even one mistake like this is one too many. The time I did go with a parent to the recovery room there were two nurses there with the child. I find it hard to believe that Matthew was left alone. But we'll have to wait and see.

Wednesday March 30, Dolphin Square

Very busy day here. Got through a lot of work. Mostly the index to Volume Four of the diaries.

Friday March 31, GOSH

A very nice young lady (Vicky) from ITV interviewed me for possible inclusion in a programme on Volunteers, with Des O'Connor, being filmed next Thursday. Whether I am in it or not I don't know, and don't much care; but what interested me was Vicky telling me that a lot of people who go into TV as a career, become greatly disillusioned after about fifteen years of struggling to become recognised, and they then give it up for, as they put it, something worth while.

I met up with Stephen (G) and his Mum Julie, sitting in the reception area by the front desk. Stephen is 10 on 16th April. He was in Louise Ward with bladder problems. I bought him some sweets. He's coming back Thursday and staying the night.

David (S), 13, in Clarence, who had hip surgery, has returned to hospital suffering from appetite loss and absencias (this is what his father put in my notebook), and to look at he is very thin and cannot take much in. On the TV there was wrestling and his father said he likes this, but if you talk to him he just looks and smiles but that's all.

Ryan (H), also in Clarence, had his legs in plaster, one plaster green, one red (they seem to go in for coloured and striped plasters now); his legs were crossed so they've been reset.

In Helena I saw little William (J), 11 months. He's a gorgeous baby with a lovely smile. He has a pancreas problem: it keeps flaring up so he's having tests. Baby Mara, with her Grandmother Kay, is still in Helena. They've been in over a year, had a short break, and are now back. Mara has a lot wrong, a lot of complications.

Kevin (G), aged 11, in Tiger Ward, who is from Aberdeen, has brain pressure. He has lost the sight of one eye and has 30% sight in the other. His Mum was with him, and they are returning home tomorrow. They were so cheerful. It's one of the many things you learn at GOSH: how courageous parents and their sick children are.

Dale (Groves) is back in Parrot. I gave him a £1 for his 13th birthday which was on 29 March.

I saw also baby Courtney who is three months (I think it was in Helena). She was smiling and gurgling and is gorgeous. Another tiny baby, Mchala was crying, so the Nurse came in and comforted her.

In Alexandra I saw A.J. who is going home tomorrow, and Nathan who is going today. Some of the nurses read Christopher's dictations, which are in this notebook, and were very moved.

Getting back to Vicky Ashmore of ITV, I see the programme with Des O'Connor is called *Year of Promise*.

Saturday April 1, Dolphin Square

I've had a very pleasant day. Went to Chalfont St Giles and had lunch with Ali and Anita. Eleanor and Toby, 2 years and 1 year respectively, are lovely children. I waited to see what the Chelsea result was (we beat Leeds 1-0) then got the 6.02pm back.

Sunday April 2, Dolphin Square

Another pleasant quiet day. Stayed in and got on with Volume Four of my diaries. I also experimented with the opening of **Vision of Glory**, Book IV in the Forsyth series. Not an easy book, but I know it will come, and will come right if I persevere, and I will.

In *Songs of Praise* (BBC TV1) this evening there was a mother whose daughter was killed when she, the mother, had a blackout driving. The mother is very religious and I am glad because it must have been of some comfort. But I don't think there's an answer. It is, on the whole, a bloody awful world.

Monday April 3, Dolphin Square

This afternoon I went for another sitting with Bill, for my portrait. He was in publishing all his life and helps me a lot. He designed the cover for my diaries, and said today that if I go on publishing them at the rate I have been, I will be 90 before I'm finished. But I really have got stuck in now, and I'm not having the same problems with Redwood Books that I had with the other people I've used.

Tuesday April 4, GOSH

Patti told me that they want me to take part in the Des O'Connor show which is, I think, going out on 1 May. So I have to be in GOSH all day Thursday for filming. It's quite fun but I've been on TV before for GOSH, and by the time the cutting is done, even if they do include you, it's only for a few seconds that you appear. Rita , who was on duty behind the front desk, was sort of upset. She's quite a cheerful person, so tends to make light of nuisances, but three things had happened:
1   She had been burgled over the weekend.
2   Her son had fallen asleep driving and crashed his car.
3   A Belgian princess (the wife of the heir to the throne) visited GOSH so Camden Council took away cars legally parked outside the hospital, belonging to parents of sick children, adding greatly to the parents' problems.
I met Amy's (S) Mum by the front desk. Amy, 16, is in the Middlesex Hospital, so I'll write to her. There was a note from Emma (U) in my in-tray, asking me to write, so I've done this. Mark was in Alexandra Ward for his check-up. In Clarence I saw Sophia (El-K), 15 (I think) who was in pain with her back. But the pain specialist doctor is seeing her Thursday. I also saw Anthony (W),12, who can't speak but smiles a lot. I think I've mentioned him before. He's a lovely boy, and so good. His legs are in plaster, strung up apart, but he never cries or complains. His Mum said he's a good example to us all. You do see the best of everything at GOSH in the midst of so much suffering and sickness. Jason (R), 5, is back. He had a kidney transplant and

has been coming into GOSH for five years, since he was a baby, which is the length of time I've been there.

The supper in the canteen was awful, the worst I've ever had, and usually I enjoy it. Thinking to help have a good night, I drank whisky and green ginger wine just before going to bed, but I had the most disturbed night with nightmares. Never again. It was stupid.

Gemma (R), 15, is in Alex. I know her of old. A very nice girl. We are going to write. I like building a relationship with the children, it helps them a lot, and their parents, and is good for me.

Very nice letter from Eddie Davis and family thanking me for the reference I gave him for his new job. I am only too pleased to have done so.

Wednesday April 5, Dolphin Square

Had a very nice French class. Anne (Rivoire) is a super teacher. All the teachers for the French classes have been good. It was such a tragedy when one of them, Olivier, aged 28, was killed in a car crash in France. He was driving too fast and hit a tree, or something like this.

Thursday April 6, GOSH

I've been best part of the day at GOSH filming with Des O'Connor. I think the programme goes out on 1 May, but, as I've said, I've had experience of TV before and by the time they've edited you are lucky (if that's the right word) to be on for more than three seconds. But it was fun to do and I was involved in quite a lot of work. Des O'Connor is very nice and he got on well with the children.

In the evening I visited some of the children: Anthony (W) and Sophia (El-K) in Clarence. Sophia took part in the Des O'Connor programme: I had to take him in to see her in her ward.

Babies Mara and William (J) are still in Helena. I spoke to Fay, Mara's Grandmother, who is hoping Mara will be able to go home soon. I saw Mark (H) in Alexandra and bumped into Gemma (R) by the front desk. She is also in Alexandra.

Jason (R), 5, who'd had a kidney transplant had gone home, so I posted him the chocolate buttons I'd got for him. Pippa (F), 14, Parrot Ward, is having a major operation tomorrow, an intercranial one which is also to do with her arteries; it is a very big one. She gave me a cuddle and I said I'd see her on Tuesday before doing anything else.

Saturday April 8, Dolphin Square

5.30am (nearly). Am leaving shortly for Manchester, for Edwin's memorial service.
8.40pm. Just got back and am too tired to write about today. I got up at 4.00am so will do it tomorrow. A most moving service.

Sunday April 9, Dolphin Square

The service at Manchester Cathedral was very moving. What looked like a temporary small altar had a large lovely coloured photograph of Edwin, of his head taken in India, I think, as he had a round red circle (a tribal mark) on his forehead. I felt very sad when looking at the photograph. On the 'altar' too were other belongings: his stethoscopes, a small tree - the kind that's controlled by wire, three red wooden juggling battens - apparently he was good at this.
Fellow students spoke of him, his exuberance, antics, learning, his love of people, his mixture of boyishness and maturity, so many aspects of his lovable character and personality. Isobel and the two brothers Robert and James were calm, whatever their feelings were; John was making a great effort to control himself. When it was his turn to quote from Bonhoeffer letters, twice he almost broke down and I didn't think he'd be able to get through it but he did.
Three Priests conducted the service and there were a lot of people. I was glad when it was over because I can't come to terms with Edwin's death - nor with the way he died. It is so unreal, such a waste as well as a loss. The family wrote this message on the inside cover of the service sheet:
A message from the family:
Edwin was part of our close-knit family. His death hit us hard, but the astonishing reaction to this loss shows that he belonged to many others as well. The effect of his death must be partly attributable to the suddenness and violence of the event in contrast to the commonplace circumstance of returning home for the weekend. There is also the apparent waste of a life that appeared to have so much to offer.
A thoroughly decent young man, Edwin was lively and compassionate. He had an original mind, which made his company often exciting, sometimes exasperating, but never dull. He was so vital. How could he die?
Questions come early in the Doubleday household and ideas are seldom left untried. Edwin was master of the unlikely angle of

attack. Where will the preposterous ideas come from that often contained more truth than the accepted norm? Our response to Edwin's death can be no other than to try to live life to the fullest extent, and our admiration of Edwin should allow us all to be a little more ridiculous, a little more compassionate, and to be a little more colourful.

We are grateful to Edwin's friends and to Manchester Cathedral for arranging this service to celebrate Edwin's life; we thank all of you for being here and we very much look forward to meeting you after the service during coffee - Isobel, John, Robert, James.

James has his first job in marketing; Robert, who won a Fulbright Scholarship has been given a place in Harvard.

Sitting next to me at the service were John's two elderly aunts. Before the service started they were passing tots of whisky to each other, from a small bottle. They said it was to keep them calm. The one next to me told me about a poem she had written about Edwin and was asked to read at the funeral. It reminded me of Christopher's funeral when his grandfather told me about the poem he had written and read.

Monday April 10, Dolphin Square

John rang this morning to say that Edwin is getting his degree posthumously. I said I'd like to go to the ceremony. John broke down again when telling me. I don't think - in fact I know - he will ever get over this. By this I mean that no one gets over the death of a child.

Yesterday evening I rang Emma (T). Her mother said she is poorly. She is covered in skin sores inside and out; now she has osteomyelitis and is in pain. She is 14, a very brave girl. She comes back to GOSH on June 14. It's not my day in, but I will go in and see her.

Tuesday April 11, GOSH

I have a new little patient in Fox Ward, Sotiris who comes from Cyprus. He is 10+, a lovely looking child; he has leukaemia. He is in privately which, his mother told me, will cost £100,000. I asked if the Embassy were paying, which happens with most of the Middle East children, but she said she's having to pay herself. She said if she has to sell her house and car it's worth it for a life. I agree, but it's a tremendous burden.

I met Rowan (V) 10+ in a wheelchair; he is coming in for a heart and lung transplant. Steven (C), 12+, left me a note to say he is back in Annie Zunz Ward. I went to see him and he gave me a lovely birthday card. His mother is very concerned over his bladder. It is natural that parents should be stressed, but the doctors and teams are hardworking and excellent. Wendy (S), 17, was back for a check-up. I missed seeing her, so will write. I've known her for a long time. She was very ill and in a lot of pain but has made good progress. Michael (C), 14 months, Hedgehog Ward, is still in GOSH. I went to see him but he was asleep and his mother wasn't there, so I'll go again Friday.

Patti told me that, including Child Health, there are 2,500 doctors, nurses and other staff at GOSH.

Wednesday April 12, Dolphin Square

Edwin's birthday. He would have been 24. I went to Great Totham. Robert met me at Witham, we collected Vassant and there were about fifteen of us for lunch. There were efforts to be cheerful, but gloom was everywhere: in the large lovely photograph of Edwin in the drawing room (the one that had been used in Manchester Cathedral); looking at an album of photographs of Edwin; talking about Edwin. How could there be anything else when the tragedy is deep in all our minds. This super young man, so caring, so lovable, so popular, so much everything that adds up to near-perfection -and it is no exaggeration to say this; such an attractive person in every way, killed so suddenly and unexpectedly in such a horrible way. After lunch I went, with John, to his grave, and put some yellow tulips there for him. We found a bunch of flowers, still wrapped, on the grave, no name, so we left them as they were. I still find it hard to believe that Edwin isn't here. It has been a miserable, rainy day.

Thursday April 13, Dolphin Square

I've had a lot of cards today. Had another sitting with Bill for my portrait. I think it's very good.

Friday April 14, GOSH

I've had a good 81st birthday. Quite a lot of cards and messages. Cards from GOSH children: Steven (C), Stephen (G), Byron (R), Gemma (R), Ben (C); also parents, and staff front desk: Salina, Judy, Rita, Inga, Emma on reception in Robin Ward. In Clarence, in Danielle's room, the family, and Lucy and Terry (nurses) sang happy birthday!

GOSH is not a sad place; it is bright, with children, unless they can't, running around, playing and happy. But there are particularly sad cases and one is Nishka (D), aged 7, who has just had her right foot amputated. She was in Clarence, crying, and in pain, but couldn't be given more morphine for the moment. I felt so sorry for her.

I met Debbie, James' (A) Mum. James, aged 8, is in Robin, having had his bone-marrow transplant. I'm not allowed in his room but saw him through the window. Debbie was sitting outside having her supper; James was on the telephone (in his room) talking to his Grandfather.

Sotiris (E) in Fox has started his chemo treatment. It's his Mum's birthday today, as well as mine. I just don't know how she's going to afford Sotiri's treatment. She isn't wealthy, not in terms of this sort of money. She said it will be £100,000, but I was told it will be more than this. I was also told GOSH are trying to get the Embassy to pay; their Government won't, so I don't know what will happen. She said she'd sell her house and car, anything, to get Sotiris well.

By the front desk I met Rowan (V), 10+, who is coming in for a lung and heart transplant when these become available (this means the death of another child). Rowan is in a wheelchair. I saw a lot more children, little Anthony in Clarence, and Alya who came to the front desk in Victoria to see me. Mehmet, having had his dialysis, was going out with his father, and they stopped to speak.

Sunday April 16, Dolphin Square

I telephoned Ali this morning. He was just taking Anita to hospital. A few days ago she fell off a ladder when it slid from under her. She fell on it and broke three ribs, one of which pierced her lung. It's a bit worrying. He said he'd ring me later and let me know what is happening. Betty and Don are going there and staying the night. Toby has chicken pox. All day (it's now 6.00pm) I've been writing letters to people who sent me birthday cards. Twenty-one thank-you letters and four others including one to Babs. Now I've got to get on with parcelling copies of *501 Days*. I'm giving these copies to members of the Phobic Society who have written for one and sent postage. I want to get rid of them as I am revising it, condensing it and hope to make it more commercially acceptable.

A birthday card from Rhoda who does all my proof-reading, was very encouraging. On the front was a photo of W.C. Fields with the words:

It's not how you play the game, it's winning that counts. And inside Rhoda had written: *Dear William - Keep on winning!*

Monday April 17, Dolphin Square

I spoke to Anita this evening. She has to see the Consultant on Wednesday. She has a liver problem and is worried. Hopefully she'll learn more when she sees him.

All day I've been parcelling up and sending out *501 Days*. I won't go swimming tomorrow, or go to GOSH early, as I want to get all the books out.

Tuesday April 18, Dolphin Square

I took another 21 copies of *501 Days* to the post this morning. That made 37 copies posted and has nearly cleaned me out, thank goodness.

2.30pm. Just going into GOSH. I've had more letters and cards here from GOSH children.

At GOSH I waved to James (A) through the window of his room. He is in isolation. Debbie (his Mum) came out and told me his blood count shows that it (his bone marrow) is taking, which is good. James is very bored; except for Debbie and his nurses he is by himself, but this has to be.

In Fox Sotiris was being very naughty, throwing a bad temper when Lynn, Staff Nurse, was trying to inject him, in his mouth, with an anti-sickness fluid but he is a very sick child. Lynn was sitting with him for ages, and I was holding his hand, coaxing him, but he kept refusing and shouting. Later I was told he had taken it. I am sorry for him. He has now lost his hair, which is a result of the treatment.

Next door I found Michael (A) who asked if I remembered him. He is 11. He has come back for more treatment and was having a five-hour infusion in his tummy. He is a delightful boy, perfect manners, a good-looking youngster (so is Sotoris), and a pleasure to be with. He wrote in my notebook:

My neutrophils are low due to infection so I'm on antibiotics and I'm here for a week.

Anthony (W) is still in Clarence. I gave him some chocolate buttons. He's a delightful boy, very affectionate and good-natured. Tomorrow they are hoping to take the plaster off his legs. I stayed on until 8.00pm and went part of the way back with Ingibjörg.

Wednesday April 19, Dolphin Square

Cleared up a lot of letters today - birthday thank-yous etc. and now I can get down to work again.

Thursday April 20, Dolphin Square

The portrait Bill is painting of me is brilliant. Full of life.
I went to the Doctor this evening, a minor ear problem.

Friday April 21, GOSH

I looked at a brief extract from *Top Hat* with Fred Astaire, and
just caught Astaire dancing with all the chorus of men in tails
and top hats doing the routine dancing. Fred Astaire is famous,
but I wondered what had become of all those in the chorus?
GOSH was very quiet, because it is Good Friday. Sotiris was
asleep. Michael was sitting up, quite sleepy, the top half of his
body naked, covered in a rash. He's been to theatre and
something that happened during the operation caused the rash.
When I went back a second time he was quite bright and
talkative, but the third time, just before I left, he said sitting up
caused acute pain in his neck (he has part of his neck bandaged
over a tube) and pain in his tummy.
In Robin I saw James who is now out of his room. He has tubes
attached to his body and is progressing well from his bone-
marrow transplant. A huge beautiful Teddy Bear came into the
hospital which I gave to him. When I saw him earlier he
mentioned a Teddy Bear I'd given him when we first met.
Because he is open to infection I gave this bear to his father,
Tony, to take home. The bear is new but, with leukaemia, the
immune system is damaged or destroyed, so one has to be very
careful of infection.
In Clarence I saw Anthony who has had his plaster removed, but
they still have to keep his legs apart. His Mum said they hoped
to go home tomorrow. I also saw Samantha (C) in Clarence. She
is a lovely girl and is always pleased when I call to see her. I
think she has a hip problem. Nishka (D) who'd had her foot
amputated, has gone home.

Saturday April 22, Dolphin Square

Ma's birthday, and we are having the usual family gathering at
The Goat in Sunbury. It's now 6.45am and I'm not going
swimming this morning as I want to go to the Post Office and
send off two copies of *501 Days*.One is for Marie Everett, Rosie's
daughter. Marie is quite amazing. She is studying for a degree
and doing well.

In Zimbabwe white farmers are being attacked and murdered. In this country Tony Martin got a life sentence because he shot and killed a sixteen-year-old burglar. There is a lot of violence.

I got back from our family lunch at about 4.15pm. It was very enjoyable. There were Sylvia, Wendy and John, Helen, Amy and Emily, Alan and Wendy, Bobby and me. We remembered Ma, of course.

Sunday April 23, Dolphin Square

I am quite clear over my writing except **Vision of Glory**. How to set about it I haven't finally decided, so the best thing is to get on with what I am clear about and experiment with **Vision of Glory** until I'm clear about this, too.

Monday April 24, Dolphin Square

Important are the diaries and, after they are published, the revised edition of **501 Days**.

Tuesday April 25, GOSH

Michael (A)
12 next week on 7 May, recently been told that the bone marrow test that was taken a couple of days ago showed results that my ALL leukaemia has changed to AML, a worse type which was upsetting for family and me.
This is what he wrote in my notebook. When I went to see him he just said he'd had some bad news and told me about it. He spoke about pulling through and I hope he does. He has taken it quite well but his father, sitting beside him, was in a state of shock. Michael will now have much more intensive treatment.

In Alexandra I saw Patrick (H), aged 6, who said I was a nice Grandfather, and I said he was a nice Grandson.

In Parrot I saw Kelly-Louise (M) who is having a biopsy; her brother Glen and parents were there, a very nice family. Also in Parrot Kristen (M), 19 months, who has fits when she wakes up. She is having an operation, the one I saw when I spent the day in the operating theatre with William , a leucotomy.

Christopher (G), aged 12, in Victoria, has Kawasaki and toxic shock + a hospital bug. It affects his skin, which has come out in bright red patches all over. He is going into isolation in Giraffe Ward.

In Robin I saw James who is improving; also saw Maria (P), aged 5, and her Mum Patricia who is expecting her second child in a couple of weeks.

Wednesday April 26, GOSH

Marie (Rosie's) rang me this morning as she wants me to sign a paper - something to do with her university degree course. I've told her to come to GOSH as I'll be there and I can do everything on the spot. She and Brian came at about 7.30pm. I read her thesis and signed her form, then showed them round some of the hospital.

Before they came I saw Michael in Fox, who has started his more intensive treatment. I saw Samantha in Clarence, also Matthew (T) whom I've known for a few years. He's had eleven operations and is in for leg lengthening. In Victoria I saw Alya and gave her some sweets. She is going home for good tomorrow. I went to see Patrick in Alexandra but he'd gone to Radio GOSH for the evening. I met Matthew (H) for the first time. He is 10, a very nice boy, and has fluid in the lung. It's his first time in GOSH.

Thursday April 27, Dolphin Square

I was pleased to get a letter, sent to Destination Way, from a trainee barrister, who had found a copy of *The Trial* in Lincoln's Inn Library. He said he found it most useful for learning the ropes and could he buy his own copy. I sent him a complimentary copy. I'm sure if I persist with my writing, even now at 81, I can succeed.

Friday April 28, GOSH

I felt so sorry for Michael in Fox. As I've said he is having more intensive treatment. Holly, his Nurse, asked him to take morphine which he had to inject into his mouth with a syringe (Sotiris had to do this with anti-sickness and refused for some time). Michael wanted to delay but eventually Holly and I persuaded him, and he did it and was violently sick. Some sickness went onto his shorts and he started to cry. Then his parents came in and we comforted him. It is a shame to see these children so ill. The treatment, which they have to have, is very severe.

I saw Samantha in Clarence. She is better, but still very weak. I gave her some more chocolate buttons. Jack (P) is back in Lion. I also met two more little patients there: Alfie (S) aged 8, who has tumours, and Matthew (N), aged 6. In Alexandra I saw Matthew (H), 10, looking a little better. His little sister, Amy, was in a bed made from two armchairs, and his Mum was there. I also saw in Alexandra, Ben (A), aged 6 who had gone down for a little walk, relapsed, and was lying in bed, not too well, with an oxygen mask.

In Transitional Care I saw Keelan and other little children. He was greatly improved and doesn't have to have a tracheotomy now. Maureen, Sister in Alexandra, told me A.J. is back on Monday and that he tells everyone I'm his best friend.

Ingibjörg was on duty behind the desk and we left together at 8.00pm. I spent some time with Joan (Fundraising Manager) getting instructions for two functions where I am representing GOSH: the Muslim Youth Association tomorrow (I've done this before) and, on Wednesday, British Telecom. I've also spoken to them before, but in London. This time I have to go to Stafford for a dinner at their training centre in Yarnfield. I enjoy these.

Saturday April 29, GOSH

I went to Edmonton Green and, as it was a nice sunny day, I walked to the Leisure Centre in Ricket Lock Road, about half-an-hour's stroll - very pleasant. I received a cheque for £4,500 for GOSH and had a nice curry supper. There were about 600 people belonging to Ahmadujya Youth Association. I met old friends as I went there once before to receive a cheque. Two charming young Muslims, Mohamad Ali and Haroon Khwaja brought me back here. It was most enjoyable.

Sunday April 30, Dolphin Square

This morning, after my swim, I went to the Mid-Surrey Golf Club, for Margaret Hamilton's retirement party. She has been there 43 years, but has diabetes, which is why she is going, although she'll come back at odd times. She is a lovely person. I saw some of the Goodwins there including Aubrey's wife, Dianna; just before that I had been looking at Aubrey's photograph on the wall with all the other past captains, and I thought of all the good times I'd had with him and his family, when he was alive; Kurt Sieger too, but he's gone, and so many others. Anthony and Pat Goodwin were there. Afterwards I bumped into Alan (brother) and he dropped me at Richmond station.

I won £10 on the lottery - very pleasing.

Monday May 1, Dolphin Square

I've had a clearing-up day, writing letters etc. At 6.05pm on Carlton they showed Great Ormond Street. I was shown walking with, and talking to Des O'Connor, and mentioning my age - 81. Alastair and Anita and Bobby rang, and a moment ago Nettie, all saying it came over well. Anyway, that's that, and I'm quite pleased it's over. I've got a very busy week.

Tuesday May 2, GOSH

Michael is much brighter - laughing and joking, but he is a seriously ill child and you can never predict the future with this awful illness. Sotiris, next door to him in Fox, looks very ill. He has lost his hair, is white and wants to sleep all the time. His mother is deeply worried. Unfortunately James in Robin has had a set-back. I didn't go into his room but Debbie, his mother, said all around one eye is inflamed and he has picked up another infection. I told her I had seen this so often in children being treated for leukaemia - lots of setbacks.

A.J. and Mark are back in Alexandra Ward. I also saw Matthew (H). Baby Emily (B) was back in Lion Ward for one night having a new line. I saw baby Liam (D), six months, in PICU. He has a reflux lung problem. Also in Lion Ward I saw Michelle (J) who has cancer of the kidney and heart. She is 10. Her father and elder sister Stephanie, whose birthday is tomorrow, were there.

In Clarence I saw Anthony (M) aged 11, whose elder sister wrote in my notebook: *condition that affects his muscles and joints - unable to use limbs to walk, feed etc. Having an operation on his back to correct a curvature in his spine.* In Clarence also I saw David (P), Matthew (T), Daniel (McC), 12, and Isaac (V), 3+, who was born with dislocated hips.

In Parrot I saw Nia, 9; also baby Charlotte (O'C), 11 months, one of twins, who is back in Fox. She had leukaemia and is back for a check-up.

In Victoria Jason, 15, with a kidney problem, wasn't too good.

A lot of people said they saw me on TV with Des O'Connor, shown yesterday.

Wednesday May 3, Dolphin Square

Today I'm going to Yarnfield, near Stafford, to receive a cheque for GOSH from British Telecom. I'm not taking this diary with me, so will write it up tomorrow when I return.

Thursday May 4, Dolphin Square

It was an enjoyable evening. I spoke about GOSH to 70 BT people who had raised £1500 for the hospital. I sat next to Jenny Arwz, the Director. Syreata also did a lot for me, and I had a very comfortable room (BT have their own hotel). The dinner was delicious. I enjoyed it very much. My taxi driver, who brought me from Stafford Station, and took me back was delightful. His name is Lascelles (not sure of spelling) and he's lived in Stafford for 40 years. He told me that he was made redundant by a factory 8 years ago, didn't want to sit doing nothing on the dole, so has his taxi. He originally came from Jamaica, is a delightful person, a happy family man.

I've had the cover from Redwood for Volume Three of my diaries. I showed it to Bill. He said they've done a brilliant job, so I telephoned Peter Holloway and said they can go ahead with publication.

Friday May 5, GOSH

Have just had this email from Byron:
Hello William
It is Byron here. Thank you ever so much for my £5 you really shouldn't have. I am sorry I missed your program because I only got your letter on the third of May and it wasn't on. I had a check-up on Friday and had such bad news. Hearts don't like to be handled and mine has swollen and enlarged and I also still have a leaky valve which if it doesn't stop then I might have to have another operation. My cousin has been rushed from Devon to GOSH last week with cancer. She is only ten and she is very poorly. So if you go into hospital soon you will find her in the Lion Ward. Mum, dad, Jade and me possibly are coming up to see her on Friday after school (the 4.20 train, so we will be there at 6.15). It has started in the kidney and into the blood stream and now reached the heart. Things haven't gone good this holiday, me and my girl friend have split up after nearly 2 years.
I have recently started work at Blooms of Bressingham, a famous garden centre and steam museum. I work in the cafe and clean tables and wash up, but £3.20 an hour is well worth it.
Anyway, thank you very much for my money. All the best
Byron.
Since then Naomi (Byron's Mum) has rung to say Byron won't be coming today (it's a psychological thing) but she and the Twins are coming. Also to say that Byron's cousin (whom I have already seen) Michelle in Lion Ward is not expected to survive.

I will be back late this evening from GOSH, so will write about the rest of this tragic news tomorrow.

Saturday May 6, GOSH

Yesterday was very busy. I got to GOSH at 2.00pm, took the cheque from BT and my expenses to Joan (K). Then I went round to see the children for whom I'd bought sweets.

Before I left Dolphin Square there was the email from Byron, and Naomi rang, so I was prepared. I went to Lion and met

Sarah (Michelle's Mum), who is quiet and very nice. Michelle was dressed but lying on her bed. Naomi said there is no hope for her, but I don't know what the situation is. I couldn't ask because nurses are very cagey when discussing this sort of thing, in fact they very rarely, if ever, do. It is dangerous to do so as remarks can be misinterpreted. Only consultants and parents can know. But it certainly doesn't look good for Michelle. It seems the cancer has spread over her body. I spent quite a time with the two of them. In the evening Nick arrived with twin sons Ross and Bruce, aged 12. So I stayed on a short while and left them as it was then getting on for 8.00pm.

In Parrot I saw, for the first time Michael (N), aged 12+, who had a brain tumour. He was asleep for most of the time. Esther, his Mum, told me it was a terrible shock when they were told what it was, as they thought it was his eyes. She told me she'd lost her father at 59 and it just seems that some families have much more than their fair share of tragedy. She is an attractive person and, like all the parents with very sick children, so courageous.

In Parrot also I saw Kelly (M) with her older brother Glen, 10+, and parents Diana and Dennis. Kelly is going home tomorrow. There was also another relative there. I said I would write and give them my Dolphin Square address, which I will.

I also saw Nia (J), 9, in Parrot who is spina bifida, and gave her the wine gums I'd promised.

In Clarence Matthew (T) had gone home and I'll post him his wine gums. I saw Robert (D), 15, in Clarence. I haven't details of his problem, but it would be orthopaedic in this ward.

Michael in Fox is brighter. When I saw him he was nursing his throat, then said it was better. I don't know how much he imagines, as in turn he had pains in his arm, then legs, then throat. But he is seriously ill so nothing can be taken lightly. James in Robin looked better, but I only saw him through the window of his room.

What upset me very much was learning from his Mum, whom I met at the anniversary service on 29 April, that Bradley (D),12, died on 28 February 1999. I didn't know this. I sent a short note but will write again.

In Alexandra, A.J. gave me a big hug and I gave him his mints, which he likes. He gave Maureen, the Ward Sister, one and me one.

I went to see Christopher (G). He is 12 and has Kawasaki and toxic shock, and is still in isolation in Giraffe Ward, but he was asleep, and I would have had to put on an apron and wash my hands entering and leaving. I didn't go in this time.

Away from GOSH I had a call from Chrissy Walker-Munro whenI got back here on Friday. She wanted to see me, as her relationship with a man she's been with had broken up. I can't be bothered with all that. My commitments are to GOSH so I said NO!

Sunday May 7, Dolphin Square

Worked all the weekend, mostly on Volume Four of my diaries.

A very interesting talk on Nietzsche this evening. I'll write more about that tomorrow.

Douglas Fairbanks Jr. died today aged 90.

Andy has just rung - 9.45pm and we are fixing an evening for dinner with him and Jane at the golf club. He said Gemma has left school and is doing exams.

Monday May 8, Dolphin Square

The talk on Nietzsche - the series entitled *Philosophy: a Guide to Happiness* - was the last Alain de Botton gave. It was most interesting for me, what Nietzsche said, that we all have a dark period, encounter setbacks and are tempted to throw in the towel. But he (Nietzsche) said suffering and failure are to be welcomed; it's an advantage to have serious reversals because for anything worth-while you have to give an extraordinary amount of effort.

What was also most interesting was that Nietzsche's work enjoyed little success in his life-time; he was out of tune with his colleagues and his books were never read.

He got up at 5.00am, which is the time I get up, and worked until midday. He had feelings of appalling loneliness. He said married people had a nest, his was a cave.

He immersed himself in philosophy. He said anything worth-while is born out of struggle and hard work. People acquired greatness and became geniuses through hard work. On TV was an example of a ballet dancer going over her routine, her movements, again and again and again, suffering pain etc., but in the end making it seem effortless. There is satisfaction at the end, and the pain is worth it. Difficulty is normal. We shouldn't give in. We can't master ingredients of happiness straight away. Perhaps, for us, happiness is to create something beautiful. There are the virtues of hardship and failure. We can all benefit from it.

Another example. A young man whose own happiness failed said it wasn't the end of the world. He's been through the worst.

Failing is horrible, but he'd come through it. He, Paul, said how could you judge success if you haven't failed? Nietzsche said it's the manner in which failure has been met, that we should look at our problems like gardeners who cultivate something ugly, making it grow into beauty. It's entirely up to us.

Envy can spur us on to compete with a rival. Hardship is a necessary evil. Life is a risky business. You have to take a chance. It's disastrous to head for the pub. Anyone who wants to be happy should never go near alcohol. Water is enough. The last thing we should do with our troubles is to drown them.

Love never ceases, but Nietzsche had grave doubts about Christianity. Put gloves on when reading the New Testament. Christianity, like drinking alcohol, may make you feel good; Christianity dulls the pain but you don't get spurred on.

Nietzsche was poor, weak, lonely. He did not deny his pain. His life was hard, but fulfilled and richer. Those addicted to comfort are small people. Abandoning comfort is true fulfilment.

That which does not kill me will make me happier.

Not everything that makes us suffer is necessarily bad. Not everything that makes us happy is necessarily good.

Nietzsche had a lot of sickness and headaches. When a student he caught syphilis. His life ended in madness. He was put into an asylum where he died aged 56.

Tuesday May 9 GOSH

I've had a long and busy day at GOSH. Last thing this evening I went to Lion Ward and saw Michelle. Byron and Nick, his Dad, were there. Byron showed me the scar from his heart operation; but he was looking well so I hope his heart will settle down and he won't need another operation. Michelle was tired and it doesn't look very good for her. I've only been told by some of the family that she won't survive; if the cancer is in the bloodstream, and has spread, which is what Byron put in his email to me, it can't be hopeful. On an odd occasion I have been told by a Staff Nurse that a child is terminally ill, but as I've said before nurses don't like committing themselves and it's unfair to ask them, unless you are a parent and then it's the Doctor or Consultant who should be asked.

James (P) was in. Liz, his mother, said she told me, but I don't remember it and hadn't got it down on my calendar. The news on him isn't very bright and he has had to come back quickly and see the Neurology Specialist. He is in pain with his left leg and he told me that a recent operation wasn't successful.

I was quite late getting back. I saw a lot of children ending up with Michelle and Byron. When I got back there was a message from John (Doubleday). I rang back and he was talking mostly about Edwin's inquest. I told him that as none of the family are going I would make notes of what happens.

Wednesday May 10, Dolphin Square

Went to the Imperial War Museum to get a photograph of *HMS Malaya* for the back cover of Volume Four of my diaries. Photographs of the ship when I was in her - leaving America after the refit, being bombed etc. - weren't all that good; but I found one taken much earlier that will do. I have written to Constance (Bibby) to see if she's got any, possibly one with Sandy. But I can use the I.W.M. one. They are so helpful, so were the M.O.D. (Ministry of Defence) and the Public Records Office at Kew. The only place that have photographs, really, is the I.W.M. It's now 5.00pm. French classes start at 6.30pm so I'll leave in an hour.

Thursday May 11, Dolphin Square

Went to Sylvia this morning. Wendy collected me at Shepperton. This morning I had a very nice letter from Tricia (C) and Matthew, GOSH, who had seen me on TV. Also an email from Salina to say Jackie , who was in charge of the front desk and got me there, has a baby girl. I was very pleased.

I've started on the disc for Volume Four of my diaries - the final corrections - and hope to send it to Peter on Sunday or Monday.

Friday May 12, GOSH

I went into GOSH early and had lunch as I had to leave early - 4.30pm - to go to Finchley Central to spend the evening with the Stapletons.

The afternoon I spent seeing the children. Michelle in Lion is about the same, looking tired. She didn't seem worse, but didn't seem any better. She's a lovely girl. Her elder sister Stephanie was there, and her father.

Then I went to Robin and saw James through the window of his room, and gave a packet of sweets to Debbie, his Mum, who said he was going through a rough patch because of his treatment. This happens with chemo. Always the painful side - ulcers in the mouth, feeling sick, but it can't be helped, it's the only way to treat this awful disease.

Michael wasn't too good. He said he was feeling a little better, but he has diarrhoea. He gets constipated and has to be given a laxative.

In Parrot Nia (J) also wasn't too good. She was lying on her tummy and was about to be turned by her father as she has to be in different positions. She is 9. In Parrot I also saw Michael (N) 12 +. He wants to sleep most of the time, but when I was there a Teacher came in and got him involved in a simple number game. Esther, his Mum, told me the good news that his brain tumour is benign, but Michael has to have another operation on Wednesday.

In day patients were Emily (S), 14, who is on crutches all the time, and Matthew (T). I didn't know I was going to see Matthew, as in the morning I had posted wine gums to him, which I'd promised him.

Two children from Transitional Care, including Keelan, were being brought out in wheelchairs to go for a walk.

The evening with Geraldine, Kevin and the children was most enjoyable. Geraldine gave me the most delicious supper. We went to the park to see Barry, who was playing football with Karl, and he looked so well. Always in the back of my mind is the awful fear that the leukaemia will come back, but Barry has been three years in remission now so I hope - I hope so much - that his is a permanent cure.

I saw Kieran, but he was on his way out to a football meeting; also Danielle who was going bowling as part of a birthday party. Barry and Karl stayed, and Kevin showed me photographs of the once derelict house in Ireland he and Geraldine had transformed into the most lovely place. The Stapletons are a delightful family - lovely children.

Sunday May 14, Dolphin Square

Yesterday I finished the disc for Volume Four of my diaries.

I watched on TV a film about the naval battle of the River Plate. What a lot of rubbish. The men never behave in the way the film shows: laughing in action, making caustic and supposedly funny remarks. In action, I know from experience, everyone is petrified. The officers and most of the men in action may not show it, but inside everyone has that awful fear that, any second, he may be blown into eternity. War is the opposite to heroic. I am not saying that we didn't have to stand up against Hitler but let's get it right: killing is squalid and ugly, not glorious. And the heroes who fight in the war can be a bloody nuisance in peace time when they are no longer of use, and in spite of the lip service paid once a year at the Cenotaph. One example was the government - I can't remember which one - trying to get out of paying war widows' pensions.

Monday May 15, Dolphin Square

Except for an hour's sitting with Bill for my portrait I've been working on Volume Four of my diaries.
Betty rang. She's got a cold which she caught from Eleanor.

Tuesday May 16, GOSH

Anniversary of Rachel's (S) death. I wrote to Debbie.
Have just got back from GOSH (9.00pm), and am leaving at 7.00am tomorrow to go to the Holocaust Museum in Nottingham with Nettie and party, so will write today and tomorrow up on Thursday.

Wednesday May 17, Dolphin Square

Spent the day at the Holocaust Centre in Nottingham. I'll write about this tomorrow, as it's now 10.15pm. Also I'll write about Tuesday's GOSH visit, and about a letter on Ma I got from Marie Everett today.

Thursday May 18, Dolphin Square

On Tuesday (last) I saw Michael in Fox. He only had his shorts on and has now lost all his hair. He's always very serious and said, in a matter-of-fact way, that his nurses had tried to get a tube down him, to help with feeding and digestion; they had tried three times and each time the tube had crinkled up on the way down, and he felt three times was enough. So some other way will be put into operation.
One youngster that worries me is Christopher (G) in Giraffe. Twice I've been to see him, but he's been surrounded by people doing things so I haven't gone in. He is still in isolation, but it just doesn't look good.
I saw a lot of other children but nothing special to report. I didn't leave until gone 8.00pm.
Today I had a lovely letter from Geraldine . She wrote: *You were so important to me when Barry was ill and still are.* They are important to me, too.
Marie (Rosie's daughter), who had been reading extracts from

my diary to Rosie, in a long letter to me, wrote: *Your Mum was always strict but fair.*

What made a tremendous impact on me was my visit to the Beth Shalom Holocaust Museum, built by the Smith family who are not Jewish, which makes the impact all the greater. It is all so well done, the museum itself and the gardens. I could write pages on it so will just mention what, for me, stood out as particularly awful.

In the garden there stands a sculpture. It is the work of Naomi Blake and is called *Abandoned*. On either side of the sculpture is engraved a biblical quotation:

Out of the depths have I called thee O Lord.

Psalm 130 V1

Wherefore hidest Thou Thy face and forgettest our affliction and our oppression.

Psalm 44 V 24

In two small gardens around the statue there are little plaques planted in the ground; on each the name of a child killed by the Nazis, and all from the same family, that of the sculptor's. They are:

Myriam Rivka 1

Shullem 1

Hava 3

Shullem 4

Berel 4

Myriam Rivka 6

Myriam Rivka 7

Fisher Efrain 11

Judith 12

Usher 13

Then there is a general inscription:

In loving memory of the Dum family who perished at Auschwitz. Roses dedicated by Naomi Dum-Blake.

In the museum are pictures that I found haunting:

That of Herschel Grynzlay, aged 17, who lived in Paris, and in revenge for what the Germans did to his parents and family, throwing them out of their homes, he shot, in November 1938, Ernst von Roth, Third Secretary of the German Embassy in Paris. This provided an excuse for Goebbels to start, in a major way, the persecution of the Jews.

Then there was the haunting picture of Tzvi Nussbraum, a young boy arrested in the round-up after the Warsaw Jewish Ghetto uprising, led by the Jewish leader, 24-year-old Mordechai

Hinielewicz-Tzui. The boy (about 12) is standing with his hands up, two Nazi thugs pointing rifles at him. The rising was between 18 April and 8 May 1943.

On the way back in the coach Nettie, whom I sat next to going and returning, asked me if I had seen the photographs of Dr Mengele who operated on Gypsy children without an anaesthetic, removing organs and experimenting, which had to be stopped for a time because the screams of the children disturbed the people living round the camp. I missed these, but I am sure I will visit the museum again, but you can only go in a party.

Nettie got me a ticket, only £18 which included a delicious lunch and tea at the musem, and coffee on the way. Sue, Nettie's daughter; and Sheila, who is a teacher with Sue at the same school, came. Also Muriel, Sue's aunt.

The journey there and back was very comfortable. Jeff, the driver, and his assistant were very nice and caring. I was lucky to be able to go.

For £50 you can plant a rose tree in the Memoriam Garden near the sculpture, and it was Sue's idea that I should associate all the love and care given to the children at Great Ormond Street with the thousands of innocents (I think it was 1,500,000) killed by the Nazis. This a good idea and I'm working on it.

This morning I went to Mr Georgeou to have my teeth cleaned etc. and saw Francine on the way in. Bobby and I are very fortunate to have him for our dentist. I am also very fortunate to have in Westminster a first class NHS Service. Chelsea & Westminster is an excellent hospital.

Friday May 19, GOSH

My thoughts are taken up with Michael. His Mum came out of his room with me and told me the very sad news that he probably won't recover. His Consultant said this. She said it is very unusual to have a reaction against the treatment and when this does happen (I assume it means his body has rejected the treatment) there is little hope of recovery. I'll just have to see what happens. Michael asked me today how Bradley died, if it was during the night or not, and I told him he mustn't identify as each case is different. I didn't know then what I know now.

Janice and Mick were in with Scott, who had been for a long operation, but the Consultant couldn't do what he wanted because a bone had grown over the particular place, so Scott has to come back and they will try again.

It's now 8.30pm and in an hour I have to walk up to the Greyhound Pub, ten minutes from here, to collect a cheque they've got for GOSH.

Saturday May 20, Dolphin Square

John telephoned this morning. He has been thoroughly into Edwin's death; seen the place where it happened, seen the Coroner and read the evidence. John thinks (in fact he's certain) that Edwin climbed through the open window of a connecting door, banged his head badly, fell out onto the line and was killed instantly. It makes sense, because Edwin used to climb up - I presume dangerously - his hospital wall and onto the roof. I heard this from his fellow students when I went to his memorial in Manchester Cathedral. Also it seems Edwin tried to force back the train doors and John was told Edwin had once shown James how to get through the doors - very dangerous.

Edwin's injuries were horrific. The side of his head where it was hit was a bloody mess; the train decaptitated him across the shoulders; only the hand was left of one arm and his leg was crushed. He wasn't run over by two trains. The second one stopped in time, not that this made any difference. I felt sorry for those who found him, and had to take away what was left of him. I'm going to the inquest on 6 June, then I'll make up my own mind, although what John has said makes sense. I've arranged to call in and see John and Isobel the Saturday I go to Wivenhoe to have lunch with Martyn and Pauline.

2.30pm. Ali rang from Wembley, and I spoke to him and Sean.

3.20pm. The FA Cup Match is being played Chelsea v Aston Villa, so I'll put in the result when it's over.

Later: Chelsea beat Aston Villa 1-0 and won the FA Cup.

Sunday May 21, Dolphin Square

This afternoon I went to the Southfields Muslim Mosque, to hear their world religious leader answer questions. I was asked to ask a question, so I asked if the Muslim concept of eternity is the same as the Christian; but His Holiness, Hadhrat Khalifatul Masih IV said he couldn't answer that, as I hadn't explained what the Christian concept is. I also asked if differences between religions on earth are resolved in eternity. I didn't hear his answer to this, as he quoted from the Koran, and I didn't get the meaning, but that was my fault. I wouldn't have bothered to ask a question but my Muslim friend, who looked after me, wanted me to. I met friends there as I had been twice before to the Ahmadiyya Muslim Youth Association, UK, for GOSH, and I was again their guest. I had a delicious curry supper and very much enjoyed my visit.

Monday May 22, Dolphin Square

Sir John Gielgud died today aged 96. One of our greatest actors. Andy Weinel's birthday.

Tuesday May 23, GOSH

Michael (A) is an unusual child. He is very grown up for his age in all sorts of little ways. I took him in two war photos from the Imperial War Museum, as he is writing on WW2 for his school - work they have set for him. When I got to the outer reception area of Fox and Robin Wards he was playing snooker with Zak's father, and he asked me to leave the photos in his room with his own father who was there. Some time later I went in to see Michael and asked him if the photos were what he wanted and he hadn't looked at them. Most boys of his age, 12, would have wanted to look immediately.

He is very fond of his parents, and when his father said he would be staying the week in GOSH, Michael said: *God help me!* We laughed. He does come out with remarks like this. Yet I remember another time, when he'd been given a morphine injection in the mouth, and he kept on being sick, and some of the sickness went on to the leg of his shorts he started to cry (as a child would); but looking back I don't think it was just the mess, I think what came out too was pent-up emotion from his worsening terrible illness. He is only a child at heart.

It is always difficult to think of a child as dying, but the Professor has told his mother that Michael is terminally ill. The sign that his parents have accepted this is that, in turns, they are staying with him all the time, helping in his room, whereas before they would be with him a lot but not necessarily staying.

Another very sad case is Amy (S), 16, in Churchill Ward. She told me she's been having constant headaches. Then I heard she'd had strokes and other problems. I know Amy as she's been in before; in fact her mother, who was pushing Amy in a wheelchair, stopped me in the corridor near the shop and said they were back in.

I saw Michelle in Lion. Byron's parents were there, and Sarah, her Mum. Michelle is being transferred to Bristol Children's Hospital tomorrow. When I first went into her room the

Consultant was there, so I returned later.

In Parrot I saw Osman (C), aged 10. He had been knocked down by a 19-year-old girl driver. His mother said she couldn't describe the pain at seeing her son lying unconscious (close to his home), his bone sticking through one of his legs. He is restless in bed but recognises people and says a few words, so we hope he hasn't had permanent brain damage.

Some of the children from Clarence - Stephanie (S) and Daniel (McC) were two I saw - were taken out to go on the big wheel. They were quite excited, Stephanie being pushed in a wheelchair and Daniel hobbling on crutches.

I saw a lot of other children, and parents, and left GOSH at 8.30pm.

Wednesday May 24, Dolphin Square

I am going into Chelsea & Westminster Hospital to have ultrasound on my legs. I don't feel ill, but I don't feel 100%.

Peter Holloway from Redwood telephoned to say my diaries, Volume Three, will arrive on Friday. I've sent him the disc for Volume Four.

5.45pm. Had my ultrasound. Lynn, who examined me, said my right leg is OK, but there's something in my left leg which is a mystery, and could be the cause of the eczema. She called in a colleague but Lynn said it was above her and I have to go back on 7 June to see her again with a consultant. Westminster NHS is very caring. Lynn said there is nothing to worry about. If there is something there I would rather know about it.

Thursday May 25, Dolphin Square

I don't know what it is, but this last few weeks I've been feeling low. Perhaps it's the time of year, the weather, age - I don't know. But I've made up my mind to pull myself out of it.

Had another sitting with Bill for my portrait. He's pleased with the way it's developing, and I'm glad as he's done so much for me, helping me with my diaries with technical advice, and designing the attractive cover. I owe a lot to him and to Rhoda who has proof-read all my books and diaries.

Friday May 26, GOSH

A major worry is Christopher (G), aged 12. He is very ill and has gone to PICU. I spoke to the family. His Grandmother said they are very pessimistic although trying to stay hopeful. She said they have discovered he has a rare form of cancer in his neck glands (I'm not sure exactly what it is - it's not Hodgkins). I saw

71

him briefly in PICU, in his room. Nurses were all round him, cleaning and dressing him. The family were in the Parents Waiting Room.There were Christopher's parents, grandmother and sister. I have grave doubts if Christopher will recover - it's very hard because we all want to hope.

Michael looked a lot better, but from what the Professor said this could give false optimism. It's always very difficult to think of a child as dying. I had this problem with Christopher (S).

I worked very late (8.30pm) and didn't get in to see Amy (S) in Churchill, which I wished I had done.

In DJW I saw Laura (T), 10; Thabassum (R) nearly 4; Timothy (G), 15 - all heart problems although Timothy has had kidney problems as well.

Zak in Fox was shut in his room as he'd picked up a bug. Sotiris doesn't say much as he can't speak much English, but he is making progress.

Baby Hollie (T) in CICU is about the same as before. She seems to be holding her own. In Helena I played with Baby Courtney (she and Hollie are only a few weeks old) and made her laugh by making noises. I also had a long talk to Thomas's (F) father. Tom had come back from Theatre in the morning so was sleepy. In the evening, the anaesthetic having given him a problem, he was on oxygen.

Saturday May 27, Dolphin Square

George Mitchener telephoned. His voice is wobbly. He said he is 94. He would like me to go out and see him, but I don't want to. He is quite well off but a mean person. He never married but had a woman friend who was devoted to him, and one day I was with him when the telephone rang, he answered it and it was her, and when he'd finished talking to her he said to me: *That's good. We're going in her car. That will save me some petrol.* If this was a one-off thing it would be petty mentioning it, but on another occasion I took Ma to see his garden (he is an expert gardener) and he made her the most awful cup-of-tea, using stale tea leaves from the previous pot. I got to dislike him. He was always cynical about marriage, saying women only want what they can get out of you, and children worship the ground that's coming to you. I don't know whether he would still think that if he saw what goes on in GOSH.

In contrast to Mitchener, I had a telephone call from Patsy Raymond. She and Peter are two of the kindest and most generous people I know. Peter's bachelor brother died leaving £5,000,000 tied up for charitable purposes, scholarships for youngsters to go to his old school, and Peter manages all this. His father was a founder member of United Dairies. He has worked for charities and is closely involved with his local theatre etc. Patsy also does a lot. Michael, their son, who has his own accountancy firm, last year sent me £1,500 for GOSH.

Sunday May 28, Dolphin Square

The weather is bloody awful. Cold and pouring with rain most of the time. I've got a sore throat so left a telephone message on their answering machine for Derek and Pamela in case they don't want me to go there tomorrow.

On the news today it said that William Hague, Leader of the Conservative Party, who lives in Dolphin Square, has promised to restore war widows' pensions. 40,000 had their pensions taken away when they remarried. So much for all this rubbish about war heroes and laying down your life or whatever you like to call it.

Monday May 29, Dolphin Square

Went to Oxted and had a lovely day with Pamela and Derek. It was sunny, and warm enough, and the lunch delicious. They have a beautiful house *The Old Vicarage* on Crockham Hill, with a large garden beautifully designed and a lovely view. They both look well - Derek nowhere near his 70th birthday which is next January. I always enjoy seeing them, and the journey is so easy. I left there at 6.09 and was back at 7.30pm.

Tuesday May 30, Dolphin Square

I often think of past incidents: most people do. And I was thinking about my visits to Eton during the war, when a boy there (I've forgotten his name) used to call me 'the Pocket Admiral'. I don't know the reason but Pip Walker-Munro told me this and I can't remember whether it bothered me or not; but the boy was killed not long after the war when thrown from his horse and his head hit a tree. And this led me on to thinking about another incident when Pip and I were walking along and a perfectly decent-looking man was passing on the other side, wearing a pair of rather loud-coloured felt shoes. When I remarked on the shoes Pip said cuttingly: *That's the best part of him*. Pip, at 25, had suffered terrible injuries when thrown through the windscreen of a car. So I couldn't help thinking that

I would rather be a live pocket admiral than a dead Etonian, and rather have worn the wrong shoes than be an Etonian with severe brain damage.

Wednesday May 31, Dolphin Square

In my French class I sit next to two very nice girls, both of whom have just got engaged; Rachel Henry assistant toy buyer for John Lewis - she has given me toys for GOSH, and Ruth Watkins who works at the Savoy Hotel. I think it is being with them I enjoy because my French is depressing, it never improves.

I've still got my bad throat but have made an appointment to see the Doctor on Friday morning. Had a card yesterday from Vera, Christopher's Grandmother, also Kevin his brother. The card was from the Isle of Wight, where it seems they usually go, and used to go with Christopher. I'm going to the cemetery in June to take flowers for Christopher's birthday.

Thursday June 1, Dolphin Square

Ben telephoned last night but was cut off before I got his new telephone number. However there was another message this morning so I rang, spoke to Mandy his Mum, then had a long talk to Ben who was 15 last month. He has cystic fibrosis, but said everything is going well. He'd been away with his Mum, and Mark his stepfather to Dubai for a ten day holiday as Mark has friends there. I said I'd go and see him later on as he said he'd like me to, and I will.

Friday June 2, GOSH

When I got to GOSH I went straight to Intensive Care, expecting to hear the worst about Christopher as all of us (me and his family) thought he wouldn't make it. To my great relief the Staff Nurse in PICU told me he'd rallied and was back in Giraffe Ward and I would be able to see him. He was in bed in a deep sleep, and I had a long talk to his family. I said I had the feeling now, that he will pull through and I hope I am right.

When I started ward visiting, Patti, Volunteers' Co-Ordinator, gave me a GOSH book on child death, but I've never read it. I do what I feel is right and I never give parents false comfort. As with Michael , whose Mum has been told there isn't much hope for his recovery, I said she has to believe this. It is much kinder to be realistic. I remember when Rachel (S) was nearing the end, her mother spoke openly about dying in front of her, because the doctors were open about it. In one case the mother told me she didn't want her child to know the illness was terminal, so her wishes were respected.

I met Stephen (C) by the main desk and he gave me a hug. His mother said he's very fond of me.

Abdul is back in Alexandra Ward but was out so I didn't see him. Little Zac, in Fox, had just come back from an operation so was sleepy. Sotiris was very active and pedalling a scooter up and down the corridor. Although children in Fox Ward have different types of the illness it is a leukaemia ward. Zac is waiting to have his bone-marrow transplant. While I was there his Consultant and team came in.

Daren (C), 15, was back in Clarence, but only to have plaster (I think it was) removed. He looked bright and cheerful. Stephanie was still there, in her wheelchair, but is being transferred to her local hospital which, of course, is more convenient for visits.

A very sad case is Andrew. For some reason I didn't get his name in my notebook (I always get the parents - Mum or Dad - to do this) so I haven't his surname. He is extremely handsome and was lying in shorts only, and is very thin. He was put in a chair and weighed and had lost (I think it was) three stone. His parents told me the name of his disease that affects the muscles. I asked his father how long he would go on for and I can't remember him answering that, but he did tell me that he had lost his other son, Daniel, aged 10, with the same disease. Another son, now 24, married and with children, is OK. I'll try and find out more when I go again on Tuesday. The parents are remarkably courageous. Andrew's mother, who was there, said she was completely traumatised when Daniel died. Danny got pneumonia which proved fatal.

In Churchill I saw Sarah (P), 16. In my notebook she wrote: *I've got a rare disease called Moya Moya.*

She's having an operation on Monday and said she doesn't like being put to sleep. Anyhow she said she'd like white chocolate buttons from Marks, so I've got her some.

Michael has gone home for a few days before he comes back for his second course of chemo.

I saw Mehmut in Dialysis; he was the only one there.

Altogether I saw at least twenty children - probably more - including Timothy (G) and Laura (T) in RBC, and baby Hollie (T) in CICU, who may be able to go to her local hospital soon.

Saturday June 3, Dolphin Square

The Chancellor is plugging equal opportunity, getting rid of the hereditary system of government by abolishing hereditary peers in the House of Lords.

Sunday June 4, Dolphin Square

All day I've been working on GOSH children's addresses. I had a lot of them and finished a big job.

I woke up with a bruising pain around my ribs. I may have been coughing a lot and strained my muscles.

Most of today, particularly on all the TV news, there have been services in remembrance of D Day, as it's the 60th anniversary and is to be the last one. A lot of nonsense is spoken about the war. We didn't give our lives that others might live. We joined up and the unlucky ones were killed, but if they'd had the choice I'm sure they would rather have lived. I would much rather be a live coward than a dead hero. Apart from the annual sentimental Cenotaph scenes, soldiers are easily forgotten. Some years ago, when I was walking along Whitehall, past the Cenotaph, on my way to Charing Cross station to see Ma, I passed a large group of Burma War Veterans in their berets and wearing their medals, waiting for the Queen to unveil the statue of General Slim. Coming in the opposite direction to me were three teenage girls, and as they passed I heard one say to the others: *Who are those funny old men?*

Monday June 5, Dolphin Square

Saw Dr Tlusty this morning. He said my feeling tired is age catching up with me, but I wonder how much is in my mind? If you let yourself go the rot sets in.

I couldn't help contrasting an item of news on TV yesterday and today, with all the old soldiers taking part in a re-enactment of the D Day landings. A record number of soldiers have deserted from and left the army. I think it is 4000.

Tuesday June 6, Dolphin Square

I went to the inquest on Edwin. The Coroner was very nice, and all the way through sympathy was expressed for Edwin, so tragic that such a young man, with so much to give, should have been killed in this way. But it was quite obvious that Edwin was to blame. He ran through the train, in and out of the doors, to dodge the crowd on the platform; the doors closed on him trapping him inside; he got stuck between two communicating doors, probably intending to jump on to the platform. A witness (I think a Policewoman) saw him leaning out towards the platform and shouted at him. The train moved into the tunnel and Edwin's head collided with the tunnel wall. If he wasn't killed instantly he would have been knocked unconscious; he fell onto the line and was run over leaving him with multiple injuries.

The verdict was death by misadventure. The driver of the train, Raymond Dietz, hasn't been able to drive since, and when he was giving evidence he broke down. John is going to write to him. Ian (Durie), Edwin's uncle, and Sarianne, his aunt, were there. Paul Major, the Coroner's Deputy, was very kind and helpful.

John telephoned this evening, and was most concerned that nothing detrimental was said about Edwin. Nothing was, only expressions of sympathy.

The Jury added to their verdict a request that the Coroner write to London Underground expressing their concern that no-one searched the train to make sure no passengers were left on the train, and that people, including important witnesses, were cleared from the platform immediately. The platform was crowded and many people, who saw Edwin's body on the line, were deeply distressed.

I went into GOSH, saw Stephen (C) who was in for the day, also had a note left in my in-tray from Freddie (C) whom I missed as I was late in. Saw Amy (S), Sarah (P) who has gone from Churchill to Parrot Ward, Michael (A), Timothy (G) who is to have a heart transplant, and Christopher (G) in Giraffe who has considerably improved and has been promised a pet python when he gets home.

When I was talking to the Mum of one child (I won't say which one) she told me her brother had committed suicide. He was an intellectual and only 32. He took tablets which didn't work, then put a live electric fan in his bath. She said her Mother never got over it.

Wednesday June 7, Dolphin Square

I had another letter this morning from John Chambers, President of the Liverpool Beatles Appreciation Society, asking again if I would help by publishing it:

Thank you for your letter and brochure about your Diarys and our write up in your new diarys using some of our old letters, apart from using them old letters could you perhaps, do some sort of present update write up on the society plus, include our address for anyone to write to us, we invite people to write to us be that beatlesfans from 9 to 90 years of age or anyone at all, / HELP / have you a copy of your TV appearance a video to send us, this has been a bad year for me, on December 26th Boxing day, i got arrested by the POLICE. at home, after two carers women from the private agency, two scally types troublemakers, caused whilst they were Drunk some upset trouble in our home with me mum and me, thank God that we had witnesses that night, one of them accused me of assault pulling her hair, totally untrue, they called the police, i had to go to court, but was eventually fully cleared innocent, as this person failed to turn up at the court, / my solicitor said if he could get legal aide which he cant it seems, then he would (SUE) this agency, it will make an exciting chapter to my CARERS story manuscript book, imagine all the CARERS 365 DAYS / my other Manuscript MANUSCRIPT STORY / BOOK possibly sometime in the future i would hope, would be my LBAS story, the untold story of the LABS years in words & pictures, our MP for our contituency, suggested we write to the liverpool city councils, chief executive to try and obtain the X Beatles official spokescompanys new address for APPLE CORPS LT in LONDON we got it off the chief executive, who got it off the INTERNET, from the Abbey Road STUDIOS London. / we have now passed on this address to our (MP) who hopefully now he will write or fax or E MAIL the EX BEATLES & YOKO and Julian Lennon, with a view to obtaining there public acknowledgment / Apprectian & Recognition / for the society and all Beatles fans everywhere, / which would be nice, when will the Diarys be published do you know, don't worry we will pay for a copy of the new book when it comes out, vision of Glory, would you autograph it for us and date it cheers. ive just written this week to the (European Court) of JUSTICE, in Luxembour, Europe, about Discrimination in wages to carers as opposed to carers in nursing homes and council homehelps, carers should get at least the minimum wage, and Backdated. i would describe myself as a novice creative writer of fact and fiction. please write back very soon, have you got a photo that you could sign and date for us cheers.

BEST WISHES & LOVE X FROM JOHN & FAMILY & NEW. L.B.A.S. Millenium 2000. CHEERS.

john james chambers.

Thursday June 8, Dolphin Square

I've worked hard today. Collected the photograph of *HMS Malaya* from the Imperial War Museum, which I want for the back cover of Volume Four of my diaries. It's very good.

Jill Prior came in to say goodbye. She and Matt are parting (he wants to go back to New Zealand) so Jill has bought her own house in Cheshire. She looks a different person, so relaxed and happy. In London she was tense, going to the doctor for shoulder pains and so on; now she looks wonderful.

Friday June 9, GOSH

Christopher is still very ill, but slowly improving. I bought him a book on snakes - lovely coloured pictures of them - and it gave him a great deal of pleasure as he is getting a python for a present when he recovers completely. I told him how Bobby kept pythons during the war, when he was an officer in the Royal Marines. He kept three in his room in Hong Kong and said his was the only room that wasn't burgled. Later he gave them to the London Zoo.

Justine (P) is still in Clarence. Children who are in since my last visit (in Clarence) are Andrew (C), 15, who has to lie flat on his tummy (his mother didn't put what was wrong in my notebook - probaby spine); also Michael (McC), 2, who has a foot being straightened.

In Transitional Care Aleema smiled at me, she can't speak properly or move her body very much, but she has improved. Little Keelan was sitting in a small chair. He is lovely. He can speak a little, in jerks, but hasn't a tracheotomy now.

Mehmet passed me near the front desk on his way out from dialysis.

In Helena I saw Stephanie (R), 11, and Katie (S), 16. They are lovely girls.

Christopher (E), 3, is back in Victoria Ward with a possible infection.

James (A), 8, has been moved to Lion Ward. He isn't at all well. He'd gone home for a few days but became ill. I said I'd take him a game. Rachel in my French class, Assistant Toy Buyer at John Lewis, gave me quite a few on Tuesday.

I saw Christopher (P), 15, being brought in by ambulance so I went in to see him in Churchill. He has come in for investigation as his eyesight has deteriorated and he's wobbly. A brain scan has shown all clear but he'll need more tests. I also saw Sarah

(P), 16, who has been moved from Parrot. She is much better.
Alex (B), 17, was also in Churchill. He was lying crying a little,
but a bit better when I went to see him later.

In Fox I saw Michael. He wasn't worse than when I saw him last
but he didn't look much better. I think he's having a bone-marrow
transplant, but his mother was told there is no hope for him. The
last time I was in Fox the Sister asked me if I'd been in touch with
Vanessa who is at home. Her leukaemia has returned and I was
told, over a month ago, that she only has three months to live. I
did write to Sue, her mother, but they haven't been in touch.

Saturday June 10, Dolphin Square

Worked quite hard. Continued with the index for Volume Four of
the diaries.

Sunday June 11, Dolphin Square

I've been feeling low these last few weeks but feel much better
now. I swam gently non-stop for over an hour this morning.

I heard a snippet on the *Today* programme. A now famous
conductor (was it Bush?) had only 54 people at his first
performance, but he persevered.

The President of Syria died suddenly yesterday. He kept his
country stable for thirty years. He was the son of a peasant. His
son has taken over as President, at 34, because the people want
stability to continue.

Monday June 12, Dolphin Square

Last night at 11.15pm a programme on BBC TV1, called *Life
after God,* investigated the nation's beliefs and attitudes in
exploring the impact of science on belief, and asked whether a
sense of the sacred is necessary to personal and global well-
being. There were quite a number of people taking part including
Chief Rabbi Sacks and Claire Rayner. As usual and as always
they got nowhere.

Wednesday June 14, GOSH

Yesterday in GOSH I saw Christopher in Giraffe. He is still a
very sick youngster but has improved. He is still in some pain.
His father told me he had always wanted to be a policeman, but
for some reason had never approached the police but had become
a postman and had been promoted. He liked the post office and
was very happy. Also that a fellow postman and an executive
were coming tomorrow (today now) to see him.

James in Lion has improved. I bought him some crisps in a tin, I think they are called *Pringles*. Christopher (S) used to like these before he became very ill, but Christopher liked the green tin. James wanted the yellow one.

Sophie (H),10, has come into Robin Ward for a bone-marrow transplant. I have a zoo book (I am a member of the Zoological Society), which she said she would like, so I'll take it in for her Friday.

Samira (A) was back as an outpatient. She is a lovely little girl and has so much wrong with her. She's had numerous operations. She wasn't feeling too well and may be coming back again, so if she does I'll see her then. I think, among many things, she had a brain tumour. I would have to look it up to be sure. In Clarence I saw Thomas (F),14, who has, among other things, cerebral palsy. By the front desk I saw Victoria (C) who had just left a note for me. She gave me a hug and a kiss. We are old friends.

In Alexandra I found A.J. who is back for a two-week check-up. In Fox I saw Michael (W) and baby Arram.

This afternoon Geraldine telephoned and asked me out for Friday evening, 30th, and I'll look forward to that. I had, this morning, posted her a copy of this month's *Roundabout,* as my letter to Suzy, the Editor, was published, in which I quoted Geraldine who said the improvements to *Roundabout* has made it so attractive and easy to read.

Behind the front desk Judy made me a cup of tea and gave me some home-made flap-jack which was delicious.

There was an email from Alistair Perriam today, saying he enjoyed the diaries but they would only be of interest to the family. I'm not so sure. A lot of people outside the family buy copies as they come out, and this morning in the shower room Ronnie Page, the Sports Centre Manager, who always buys a copy, said he found them very interesting, and he spoke about the views I had on life after death when a young man, and asked me what I felt now? (Not much different actually).

Last week Rachel , in my French class, gave me two large bags of toys for the children.

Getting back to Geraldine , she told me she is worried that Barry (now in remission from leukaemia) isn't studying seriously enough. Barry told his mother he wanted to be a carpenter. Geraldine, a committed Catholic, told Barry that Jesus was a carpenter, but Barry said Joseph was the carpenter. I can't remember at this moment whether Jesus was or wasn't.

Thursday June 15, Dolphin Square

2.00pm. Just off to the Royal Mid-surrey as Andy, Jane and possibly Gemma, Ali and Anita, are coming for dinner. I'm very much looking forward to it. The weather is warm and dry.

10.40pm. The evening was a great success. We all enjoyed it immensely.

Friday June 16, GOSH

Went to Chelsea & Westminster Hospital to see Mr Nott, the vein Consultant. He said my legs are OK and nothing needs to be done. Mr Nott is much younger than I thought.

Christopher is much better. Quite bright and much more communicative. He wants a book on cats. He is still very ill but greatly improved.

Scott was in for a check-up and I had a long talk with Janice, his Mum. Scott has grown quite a bit. I don't know how much he takes in; he seems to respond with his eyes and expressions.

Nicholas's (C) Mum left me a note to say his leg frame wasn't successful and he may have to have an amputation. I'll write to her and to Nicholas..

I gave A.J. in Alexandra a toy and his £1.

It was Sophie's (H) birthday. She is due for a BMT in Robin and was having a party in the playroom with lots of other children. I gave her a zoo magazine as she likes animals.

In Transitional Care I saw little Keelan who has improved a lot, and even says a few words. Marc (L),14, is back in Clarence. He has so much wrong with him and has had so many operations. He is very polite and courageous.

Saturday June 17, Dolphin Square

Went to Wivenhoe. Martyn and Pauline took me to lunch at the *Black Buoy*. Very pleasant. Then I went on to John and Isobel. At Totham Robert met me and we called in at the local church. I could have gone to a barbecue but had a sandwich and beer and came back. James was there having finished his exams in Cambridge. All the family are trying to come to terms with losing Edwin but it's very hard. Isobel said, very sadly, that it's awful to think we will never see him again.

In the train I found today's paper which had an interesting article on *Westlife*, the Pop Group of delightful youngsters who came to GOSH. I'll write about it tomorrow as it's getting late - 10.30pm.

Sunday June 18, Dolphin Square

In the paper, writing about *Westlife*, it said some may think being a member of a successful Pop Group one of the most glamorous jobs in the world, but recently the Irish youngsters have been suffering the effects of a punishing schedule. One collapsed after a radio performance, flew home, and said it was all too much. *Westlife* is already the most successful band in British chart history and last year had a collective income estimated at £14.3 million. Other members of the band are reported to be feeling the strain. They are off on planes every day. They are very professional and keep smiling. When I met them at GOSH and spoke to them I found them delightful. Last week (I think it was) the anniversary of one our most famous Pop stars was celebrated. I can't think of his name right now, but a year ago he hanged himself. Nothing is ever as it seems.

Nettie rang me and asked if I could go for lunch, as she was entertaining American friends and someone pulled out at the last moment. I went, had a delicious lunch, and met Loren and Carol Geistfeld. He is Professor of Economics at Ohio University; he has taken a copy of *The Trial* back for the law library. They are a charming couple.

Monday June 19, Dolphin Square

This afternoon I had another portrait sitting with Bill . He is quite pleased with it, so am I.

It is so hot and close at the moment, but there is a promise of cooler weather.

Tuesday June 20, GOSH

Emma who now works in Robin/Fox reception, told me today that little Ryan is at home in a coma and could go at any time. I knew, some time ago, that he has a severe leukaemia and is terminally ill. I think he is 2+. A few days ago Emma told me that Ryan's little brother, Joe, 15 months, was rushed into hospital with meningitis and died the same day. Ryan's Mum is pregnant and, as Emma said, it is just appalling to think what that family has suffered.

I saw Christopher. He is looking much better but is still very ill. But he is responding now, and as he was very near to death only weeks ago, it is remarkable. I gave him the book on cats I had.got for him. He was very pleased.

Michael seemed about the same as before. I also saw little

Stanley in Fox Ward and Dorfana who wasn't too well. I gave Marc (L) the mints I promised him. He is having another operation on Thursday. I also saw Andrew (C) and said I'd take him some lead toys which Rachel gave me.

In Helena I gave Katie (S) the chocolates she asked for, and in Alexandra I gave A.J. his mints and £1.

Near the front desk I met Charlie (W), now 2, running around. His Mum, June, said it cheered her up when I went to see them when Charlie was in GOSH, as a baby, with leukaemia. She said my visits meant a lot to her. Many parents have told me this.

This evening I saw a documentary on the Channel Islands when under German occupation. Even after all this time I still find it hard to believe that a supposedly civilized race could be so continually barbaric. The programme was about (mostly) a hero called Albert Bedane who saved the lives of the persecuted at great risk to himself.

Wednesday June 21, Dolphin Square

I had a delightful email from Margaret (H), whose son, David, was in GOSH in March. He'd been so ill, having had bladder cancer when he was 3. When I saw him he was nearly 11. GOSH built the little boy a new bladder from his intestines. Margaret said GOSH saved David's life, and he is now at school taking part in all activities - marvellous.

Thursday June 22, Dolphin Square

Went to Bexhill and had a delicious lunch with Peter and Daphne Studd. Peter told me they had destroyed all Maud's personal possessions, photographs etc. They gave Bill's RAF uniform to a charity. I didn't know, until Peter told me, that Maud had had so much tragedy. Her mother, when pregnant, fell on ice or something like this, and died when Maud was 6. Her brother shot himself, the other brother was killed in Egypt in WW2. Something went wrong with her father, but I can't quite remember what. Tom, her husband (whom I knew), died of cancer and she lost Bill aged 19. Bill wasn't even killed in action. His engine packed up because a mechanic had left a fault there and Bill crashed into a field, and into some trees, in Scotland. Maud was such a wonderful person, staying on top of all this; I think because of her Catholic religion. She died aged 84, about this time Peter said. She rented the top flat in his place. I would like to have had Bill's uniform, but I have his letters. Maud is the only person who left me money in her Will. It was £500, a lot in those days. I was very touched and used the greater part of it to buy my Hewlett Packard printer in memory of her. I hope she and Bill are reunited.

Saturday June 24, Dolphin Square

Yesterday I went to Shenfield where Vera, Christopher's Grandmother met me at the station. We walked to the cemetery where I put flowers on Christopher's grave for his birthday on Sunday when, had he lived, he would have been 11.

I had some very sad news, that baby Mara (G), who had been in Helena for over a year, died at home. I will write to her Granny, Fay who was with her a lot.

Yesterday also, I had a long talk to Ingibjörg (Andrews) in the Italian Hospital (it belongs to GOSH and is used for fundraising etc.), where she now works behind the reception desk on the ground floor. We discussed **Vision of Glory** and the form it might take. When I was walking along to see her I met Hanna, her daughter, who is a top model, a beautiful girl with a lovely personality.

Getting back to Shenfield. In the cemetery, not far from Christopher, is a stone, still with the inscription clear, of a 3-year-old who died in 1969. The grave had been neglected. Vera thinks the parents may have died. Anyhow she tidied it up and put in a plant. I thought this very kind as it means the child is not neglected. Vera is a very kind person.

Sunday June 25, Dolphin Square

Today is Christopher's birthday. He would have been 11.

Monday June 26, Dolphin Square

Stayed in and worked. Had a sitting with Bill this afternoon.

Tuesday June 27, GOSH

A very sad day. Michael has been given about six weeks to live, unless a drug coming from abroad works a miracle, which is unlikely. I saw him about three times: the first he was lying near the window, his tummy bare and he was rubbing it, it is very swollen; the other times he was sitting on the edge of the bed, pale, weak, not speaking a lot. He has lost all his hair. I find it quite stressful and can only hope, like his mother, that a drug that's coming from abroad for him, works; but it doesn't look good. He is only 12.

Christopher (G) has come into Fox Ward. He was making such good progress but has had a stroke, paralysing his right side. That is now returning to normal but he can't hear. He was rushed into PICU, but what frightens his mother is that he may have another, and more severe, stroke.

I saw other children, and one parent said: *Keep up the good work.* Of course I will go on with what I'm doing for as long as I can, but it is not easy.

The other sad news is that Nurse Nina told me Vanessa died and her funeral was (I think) last weekend.

Wednesday June 28, Dolphin Square

Ben telephoned this evening. He was in Brighton Hospital for an operation to relieve a blockage. He sounded very cheerful. I said I'd go and see him in July. He hopes to leave hospital tomorrow.

I sent the back cover design for Volume Four of my diaries to Peter.

Friday June 30, Dolphin Square

I'm going into GOSH this morning and hope to see Michael who is due in Elephant Day Care at 11.15am. And I want to see Christopher and others. I'm leaving at 4.30pm as I'm spending the evening with the Stapleton family in Finchley. I'm very much looking forward to it. I'll write about this tomorrow as I won't be back until late.

Saturday July 1, Dolphin Square

I had the most lovely evening with Geraldine and her family. Kieran went out, so did Danielle and Barry. Karl stayed in with Geraldine, Kevin and me and we talked about all sorts of things including, of course, Barry's health and the wonderful way in which he has fully recovered from having been so ill. I had a delicious meal, salmon and salad and strawberries. Geraldine is going to their house in Ireland for the summer.

Before going out there, in GOSH, I went to see Christopher who had just had another stroke. The Doctor was with him testing the bottom of his feet, his hands, and so on for a response. Christopher wasn't responding well, although he had slightly improved when I called back just before leaving. It is very worrying.

I had gone into GOSH early as I was leaving early to go to Finchley, and was expecting to see Michael in Elephant Day Care where he was due at 11.15am. But I was told Michael had been rushed into his local hospital (I think it's Croydon), and I have the feeling he's near the end. It's very, very sad.

Monday July 3, Dolphin Square

The year is going by very quickly.

Tuesday July 4, Dolphin Square

Shabnam (M) had left me a note in my GOSH in-tray to say she'll be in today, so I rang her in Victoria Ward and said I'll write. She'll be in again on 20th and although it's not my normal day, I'll try and get in to see her.

Wednesday July 5, GOSH

Michael died in his local hospital. It is always very distressing to lose a child, but particularly so with Michael, as he was extraordinarily mature for his age. When I last saw him in GOSH he was sitting on the window seat between his parents, and his father, William, was stroking his back gently. Michael looked pale and ill, and was a little unsteady. We knew, and he knew I'm sure, that he hadn't long to go. Today I was talking to a Staff Nurse and she said Michael was very advanced for his years, and that he did know he was dying because over the weekend, the last couple of days of his life, in his local hospital, he refused all drugs, and would allow no visitors, not even his brother and sister and he died Monday morning.

Little Ryan was buried today alongside his 15 month-old brother Joe.

I don't hold out much hope for Christopher who is now in Fox Ward. He was making such good progress but has now become very ill. I hope he pulls through but it is very worrying.

11.45am. I was looking through my GOSH notebook to get Michael's home address and I saw that on 18 April he had written:

My Neutrophils are low due to infection so I'm on antibiotic, and I'm here for a week.

A little farther down, on 25 April, he wrote:

Michael A.

12 next week on 7 May. Recently been told that the bone marrow test that was taken a couple of days ago showed results that my A.L.L. leukaemia has changed to A.M.L., a worse type which was upsetting for Jin-Hua (his nurse) and me.

Thursday July 6, Dolphin Square

I kept thinking today about Michael and little Ryan, but particularly Michael as he was older, and I was with him a lot more. It is hard to believe he has gone so suddenly, although it was expected. I have written to his parents.

Friday July 7, Dolphin Square

In the swimming pool I spoke to Stuart Sampson, a leading lawyer in the CPS. He told me he went to a memorial service for a barrister friend who had recently taken silk (become a QC), so was at the beginning of a career full of promise - he would probably have become a Judge. He was only 50 when he got cancer and died.

8.50pm. Just got back from GOSH. Met Christopher's Mum in the Peter Pan cafe. He is very ill. He'd been to theatre and the cancer has spread to his brain, which was the probable cause of the stroke. Will write more tomorrow.

Spent the afternoon with Rhoda.

Saturday July 8, Dolphin Square

I got up late (for me) this morning, as some damned girl about two floors below had music blasting out at 2.00am. When I got down there Security were sorting her out. I told her that her behaviour was disgusting. It took me quite a time to get to sleep again.

Yesterday I didn't go in to see Christopher. His mother said he isn't really with it as his hearing has gone, and I don't think he can speak properly. There is a photograph of him pinned up on the wall of his room, showing him before the illness, well built; now he is thin with awful rashes and lumps over him. I don't think he will pull through; I think too much is stacked against him. I would like to be proved wrong. His mother is very distressed, naturally.

I saw other children. I do find that children dying is emotionally punishing, as it is a loss, each time, and the child stays with me. But it is part of my job.

As I wrote yesterday I saw Rhoda and we had a long talk, an hour-and- three-quarters. I always enjoy my visits.

I hardly ever buy a daily paper, I'd rather see the news on TV, but in today's *Times* there was an article on Glenn Waddington, a young entrepreneur, who grew up on a Huddersfield council estate, was teased as a child for not being able to afford shoes, then turned an £800 bank loan into a £5 million company, becoming one of the leading bathroom suppliers in the country. Aged 24 he suffered a brain haemorrhage after complaining of feeling unwell at work and going home to rest. He was found dead in his bath. He gave many people opportunities because he wanted them to share in his success. His funeral took place yesterday at Kirkheaton Church, Huddersfield. He leaves a fiancee, Kirsty.

Sunday July 9, Dolphin Square

Bobby said yesterday, on the telephone, that one reason my diaries appeal to people, is that the majority can identify, because most people are full of resolutions they don't keep.

Went over to see Sylvia. Wendy collected me at Shepperton. It was a lovely sunny morning although it's been pouring with rain the rest of the day. John was there, cutting the hedges. The garden looks beautiful. There are plants there which brother John put in. We still miss him a lot.

Had another sitting with Bill. I told him Sylvia had said that what she liked about the diaries is that outside events are mentioned. Bill said the sad thing is they will come into their own, as social history, after I'm dead. Inga said the same thing.

Tuesday July 11, GOSH

Tom Gavin came to GOSH for supper. I took him to Clarence. A Gambian boy was sick so we looked after him until the Nurse came and then Tom had to put on an apron and help the Nurse. He was very good. Then we went to Fox. The Nurses took Tom into their sitting room while I saw Christopher. He is still very ill; his skin is bright red, he had blisters and rashes on his leg, he is restless and moans a lot. Poor boy, and his poor family, parents and grandparents who are with him all the time. I don't hold out a lot of hope for him, but I hope I'm wrong.

I saw little Yasmin in Alexandra. She was lying with her head inside a square glass oxygen container. She is lovely, a pretty little girl and very bright.

Wednesday July 12, Dolphin Square

Email from Tom Gavin saying his visit to GOSH was an amazing experience and he'd got a lot out of it. He was particularly affected by the courage of parents and their sick children. This has always affected me in the same way. Tom read what some of the parents had written in the chapel book; no-one could read these without being greatly moved.

Thursday July 13, Dolphin Square

The weather is bloody awful. Miserable, raining, chilly.

Friday July 14, Dolphin Square

Patti said a lot of people who come to GOSH ask if I'm there, so it would be helpful if I could let them know the days that I am in. Up to now I've been going in Tuesday and Friday afternoons and evenings, but from now on I'll go in one day a week, but for the whole day and see how it works.

I saw Christopher twice. He is very, very ill. He has come out in huge blisters all over his body, which are being pricked and drained of fluid. His skin all over is bright red. He is under sedation with morphine. The Doctor came in the second time I was there and they are going to try a pill that has a small percentage of valium. They can't give too much morphine. The family, parents, grandparents and aunt, who are with Christopher are under enormous stress. Christopher's father had to lie down twice with migraine.

Zak's father gave me some lovely photographs of little Zak, who is getting into remission from leukaemia; he also gave me one of Michael taken, smiling, with one of the Spice Girls (I think it's Geri Halliwell). Michael died about two weeks ago. I miss him a lot, as I do all the children who have died.

Little Samira (A) is back in Parrot Ward. She is so bright and cheerful. She has wires plugged to her head and chest for investigation. She is amazingly bright and cheerful, so are her family. She's had thirteen operations. She is so pretty with a lovely personality.

While I was standing near the volunteers' desk Kristian (P), now 13+, came over with his father. I've known Kristian for all the years I've been in GOSH - he's had leg and knee problems - so he would have been about 8 or 9 when I first knew him. He is very good-looking with a quiet, pleasant personality. It was nice seeing them again.

I get quite a lot of letters from children and parents. I have had four + a card this week.

Sunday July 16, Dolphin Square

The work in the wards has grown enormously, which is why I want to try coming in for the whole day. Also I have built up a large correspondence with children, and often parents as well. They telephone and write to let me know when they are coming in; and if it's a day I am not in at least I can keep in touch. I have found this means a great deal to them.

This last week I had a letter with £5 for Laura (B) from her Mum to get flowers in the chapel for the anniversary of Laura's death on Friday. I had a card from Emma (U); a letter and drawing from Nicholas (C) aged 7; a letter from the Mum of a boy recovered from leukaemia; a letter from the Mum of Bradley, a boy of 13 with special needs, and she also enclosed a photo of him; also four messages to say that Victoria is coming in on 18th, Shabnam on 20th, Scott on 25th and Adam on 28th. I will be in for Shabnam so will be writing to all the others today. Most weeks are like this.

Tuesday July 18, GOSH

I went into GOSH today for a reason that I will come to later. I saw Christopher who is now in intensive care on a life-support machine. His grandparents were with him, then John and Jackie came in, then Jackie's sister. The lady Doctor came in while I was there. Two Nurses were looking after Christopher, doing various things all the time, but it seems his life-support will be switched off and that will be the end. It is very, very sad. He is lying there naked except for a sheet over half his body, his face to one side, a tube in his mouth and wires attached to him. Terrible for those watching.

I'll be going in again Thursday, but whether he will be there or not, I don't know. Such a contrast between his thin body lying on the bed, his eyes closed, breathing heavily to the photograph of the handsome youngster that was on the wall of his room in Giraffe.

Why I went into GOSH today was to get my face photographed. I had a nasty fall, tripped over a jutting pavement slab in the gardens here; my face is completely black and blue over one side. I also had another tumble in the afternoon, as I put on dark glasses to hide the bruising, so can't see properly, tripped over a car post (also in the grounds here) and fell on my shoulder. I had the photographs taken in case I decide to make a claim.

Wednesday July 19, Dolphin Square

I had such a bad night aching all over, but it's eased a bit this evening.

It's been a perfect summer's day, warm with a gentle breeze, and so lovely in the country where I have been to have lunch with John and Isobel. Robert was there when I arrived. After lunch Isobel cut some flowers and we took them to the cemetery for Edwin's grave. Isobel had a short weep and I felt very sad, so did John of course. Close by was the grave of another young man of 23.

I enjoyed seeing Isobel and John and Robert. I always do.

Thursday July 20, GOSH

Christopher died.

Before I went to GOSH I met Derek Collins at Victoria Station and gave him some MCC wine, which he wants to auction in aid of his cricket club.

At GOSH I learned the sad news about Christopher.

Shabnam had left in my in-tray a beautifully framed picture of three tigers. I saw her before I left and thanked her. I also saw Emma (T) who looked better than I've seen her for a long time. I'll write more tomorrow as I am tired. It's just gone 9.00pm and I've been on the go all day.

Friday July 21, Dolphin Square

I was quite touched. I had a get-well card from all my friends in the Marks Pantheon food store, from Kathy and the girls who work there. Also a get-well card from Margaret.

Karl (Stapleton) telephoned me this morning and told me he was soon off to play football. And I spoke to Barry and Geraldine.

I still have very heavy bruising all over my face. My ribs are not so sore but a bit painful in bed.

Mike Newland, my doctor friend rang this evening. He's not so good. He has cancer of the prostate, heart problem and arthritis in his knees. He's ten years younger than me and amazingly cheerful.

I'm working on Volume Four diary proof today. I'm taking this week off because of my fall so hope to finish it soon.

Nettie rang to say Michael Collins her son-in-law will buy John's Bowra maquette sculpture. He has always wanted it and John will put the money into Edwin's memorial fund, which is to pay for medical lectures in memory of Edwin.

Sunday July 23, Dolphin Square

Downstairs this evening I met Celia with her son Irving who is a solicitor. Irving doesn't do personal injuries but he was very helpful over my fall. Lee, Celia's 14-year-old grandson, whose bar mitzvah I went to, was there, also Rene, Celia's sister. They are very nice.

My bruising seems slightly better and my ribs don't ache so much.

Monday July 24, Dolphin Square

Had a letter from Leon, my friend who is an Auschwitz survivor, and whose wife and child were murdered by the Nazis there. Leon wrote:

My little boy Barney will live on in name. A friend of mine, he is a solicitor, has named his second son after my son, what an honour! So Barney lives on in name and memory, he is now four - five years young but later his parents will mention him about me (funny how God deals with people).

Very touching. Barney was four when he went to the gas chamber. Leon will be 90 next birthday.

An idea came to me today to write **Vision of Glory** through letters to different people, not to the same person. Anyway, I'll experiment.

Tuesday July 25, Dolphin Square

Rhody Fletcher my next door neighbour is lonely, which is understandable. I'm quite happy as I am, with my writing and my many GOSH children.

Wednesday July 26, Dolphin Square

Nettie has been very helpful. She put me in touch with a top solicitor who said unless my eyes had been affected by my fall, I wouldn't get enough to justify litigation. If my eyes are OK (I'm going to Moorfields Friday and I hope they are) I won't make a claim. It's not worth all the trouble of getting a medical report etc.

Thursday July 27, Dolphin Square

I went to Paddington to see where they have put John's Brunel Statue in the reconstructed station. It's not in the central position now, but in the little square off platform 1 where the taxis arrive and leave. It fits in, but is not prominent any more, and it's quite dark there compared to the rest of the station.

My bruising is clearing up. I felt a bit lethargic this afternoon but got on with some work on the proof of Volume Four of my diaries.

Saturday July 29, Dolphin Square

Some of us from GOSH, Rita, June, Millie and Peggy went to the Isle of Dogs (Island Gardens) and had lunch with David and Judy Longbottom (Judy has just retired from the GOSH front desk). The lunch was delicious, the day sunny and warm. Most enjoyable.

This evening there was a message from Ben who is in Alexandra Children's Hospital, Brighton. I'm going to see him on Wednesday.

Sunday July 30, Dolphin Square

I've had another delightful day. Went to Boreham Wood where Richard Leslie my godson is Vicar. The service was excellent, the church packed. His family were there: sister Mary, Victor (husband) and daughter Vanessa from America; sister Clare and Fitz, also Christopher (Richard and Jenny's son), and Jenny of course. After the service we had a lovely barbecue in the vicarage garden. Another lovely sunny day.

This evening I spoke to Ben in Brighton who said he's got his Mum's permission for me to take him out on Wednesday.

Sylvia rang to see if my bruising had cleared up, which it almost has. And my ribs, though still a little achy, are better.

Monday July 31, Dolphin Square

Went to see Mike Newland my doctor friend today. He is very helpful with advising me on medical problems. He said life for me is well worth living because I have so much to do; I have a strong reason for going on living and after I'm dead I won't care. He said I should have tests now and again (the recent ones were all clear) and relax. It's no good worrying about getting cancer or having a heart attack; worry may make it more likely to happen. Just hope I can finish all I want to do. If I have little symptoms I should tell him and he will explain them, and he would tell me if I should take further action. Cancer is inoperable if you leave it too long. Relax. Don't wait for things to happen. **RELAX.**

Tuesday August 1, Dolphin Square

I had drinks this evening with Rex and Dickerle Boys. I got Rex talking about the Burma War where he was an airforce pilot. He was shot down and then taken up a river by the Burmese, with the enemy on either side. Later he was in hospital in Burma when the Japanese arrived. They murdered the doctors and nurses and went round bayonetting the patients, but Rex escaped through a window. He is now 85 (I think), has cancer which is controlled, a leg very damaged so he has to wear a brace and other support. He is incredibly brave, so is Dickerle who isn't well. They are cousins, have been married for 33 years although both were married before - Dickerle twice, but her husbands died. A very brave and charming couple.

Wednesay August 2, Dolphin Square

Just come back from Brighton where I took out Ben who is in Brighton Children's Hospital. We left just after 2.00pm and got back at 7.00pm. The weather was sunny and warm, but windy. We had a wonderful time, walking along the front and on the pier where Ben went on various things - I joined him on one, circulating fast cars, which was scary for me. He went on a lot of these including dodgem cars. He played some machines and won prizes. I bought him a model kit and "How to learn 250 card tricks", and we finished in a pizza restaurant. He enjoyed it, so did I.

I came back to some sad news on my answering machine from Albert Chick's son, to say that Alby died yesterday. Rang and spoke to Janet (daughter). Alby collapsed in a coffee shop in Victoria Street from a heart attack and died instantly. He'd been suffering from angina for some time. It was Steve who rang me. Brenda (Alby and Doll's other daughter) lost her husband a year ago. I think he was about 50 and had cancer, but am not sure. Very sad.

Thursday August 3, GOSH

Bobby is 80 today.

I started my new GOSH routine, which is to go in on a Thursday for the whole day. It means I can go round all, or most of, the wards. I've been away for ten days because of my two falls.

A.J., Louis and Abdul were back in Alexandra. While I was away, Sotiris in Fox had been rushed to Intensive Care but is better. Laura (T) is back in DJW. I saw Mehmet and Jason in Victoria, Michael and Freddie in Dialysis and others.

I wrote to Ben in Brighton.

I also saw Scott with Janice and Mick in Parrot.

Friday August 4, Dolphin Square

I was thinking today about Ben. He is such a delightful youngster, a charming personality and mature. One can only hope that progress is such that a cure can be found for him.

Saturday August 5, Burley, Hampshire

Arrived here this afternoon to stay with Betty and Don. Glorious sunny weather. Sat outside this evening. Very peaceful in the beautiful secluded garden, the New Forest all round.

Sunday August 6, Burley, Hampshire

It's 5.45am and I've come down and made myself a cup of tea. Betty and Don are still in bed, and I'll go back to bed when I've had my tea. It's light outside and very quiet and peaceful. The change here will do me good. It's the travelling I don't like, crowded trains, noisy people especially now these awful mobile phones are the rage. In Brighton, talking to Ben, who has one, I thought of getting one, but on the TV news yesterday a Doctor is suing a mobile phone company for huge damages, as a tumour in the brain, which has made him terminally ill, was caused by a mobile so he says. There is no proof mobiles damage the brain, but there is no proof they don't, so I'm not getting one. I'll go on with this later, as this afternoon we are going to Lyndhurst to see Andrew and Helen Perriam and the two children in their new house in Lyndhurst.

I went into the village shop this morning and got some cards, and for the first time read the inscription on the village war memorial. The smarmiest inscription of this nature that I have seen. It read:

In memory of those who went out from Burley and fell gallantly in defence of their country in the great war 1914-18. "Their names liveth for evermore"

Erected by Col. Frank Willan and his wife as a token of their gratitude to God for the preservation of two sons and a son-in-law in the army who served in France during the war.

There were twelve names of officers and men from the First World War, and twenty officers and men including a naval chaplain and midshipman from the Second War whose relatives were unable to express gratitude to God.

We went to Lyndhurst and had tea with Andrew and Helen. Their new house is very nice. There is a field at the back and a lovely view over the New Forest. Joe and Emma are lovely children. It was very enjoyable.

Monday August 7, Burley, Hampshire

Nearly 8.00am. Am sitting downstairs with a cup of tea. Don and Betty are still upstairs. I'm returning to London today. The break has been good for me. I've been working on the best approach for *Vision of Glory* and I think it could be in the form of a letter, because one thing I am good at is letter-writing. Frank Jackson said several times that if I could go over and over, again and again, getting a letter right I can do the same with my other writing. I just feel that I must make a start on *Vision of Glory*, because if I don't write anything, I've nothing to alter.

What I have in mind is writing a letter to James (a fictional character) and somehow revealing my life, and my thoughts through others; also making use of all the notes on various things that I have written over many years. My trouble is I have so little confidence in myself, and it's hard to overcome, and for me it is a miracle that I wrote *Violence*, the one book I'm more than happy about and, whatever the criticism, I wouldn't want to alter in any way.

In the train

I've just got on the 11.00am at Brockenhurst. I've managed to get a seat. There is a nice quiet man sitting opposite, but a little down on the left are a noisy crowd of women constantly laughing loudly and in a seat near them is a screaming child. How I hate all this, even if it is a part of life's rich tapestry. This is what I dislike about going away. Even Scotland, when I go first class, is dreary. And this day and age there are constant interruptions from people using mobile phones.

Dolphin Square

I went into GOSH, had lunch, and saw Janice and Scott.
Ben is having his operation tomorrow in Brighton Children's Hospital. I've got a Burley card to send him.
 I found letters from Sam and Nicky Cole in my in-tray. Nicky has to have his leg amputated.
Alec Guinness, who unveiled John's Charlie Chaplin statue in Leicester Square, died aged 87. Also Robin Day who was 76.

Tuesday August 8, Dolphin Square

7.10pm. I've been telephoning Brighton Children's Hospital to see how Ben is. He is in Intensive Care after his operation, but the lines are busy so I'll have to try again.
I've started on *Vision of Glory*. I must keep going now. I don't concentrate nearly enough, but that's the old, old story.
I got through to Intensive Care but I couldn't get a clear

picture on Ben, only that he's in the process of recovering. I'll try again tomorrow.

Wednesday August 9, Dolphin Square

I went to Alby Chick's funeral. He is buried in Wandsworth Cemetery. Doll, his wife, said they were walking to Victoria Station, saw me, and tried to catch up. I was returning from Marks & Spencer. Shortly afterwards Alby collapsed and died. I wish I'd seen him. I went to Wandsworth then back to their flat, saw son Steve, who is so nice and the image of his father. Of course all the family were there.

Alby is buried near Brenda's husband who died quite young, not long ago. Alby was 73.

I telephoned Brighton Children's Hospital. Ben is feeling fine.

Thursday August 10, GOSH

I gave A.J. in Alexandra the allowance I make him while he's in GOSH. I also gave him the mint assortment he likes. He is very fond of me, as a lot of the children are, and I am very fond of him and them.

Baby Natasha is back in Fox. Unfortunately her leukaemia has returned. Very worrying. Sotiris was on top of the world as he's going home for a few days.

Charlotte (T) is back in Clarence. She is 16 and when she saw me in the reception area she came over and kissed me. I also got a hug and a kiss from Victoria (C) who was in Alexandra in the next room to A.J.

I saw Laura (T) in DJW. They've got her heart right but she has other problems.

Iris had telephoned to say she would be in Dental with Sean, so I saw her there at 2.00pm and sat with her until she left with Sean about three quarters of an hour later. He still has epileptic fits but his teeth are OK. He is 16 now and is in a wheelchair all the time. He's a good-looking youngster and has such care and devotion from Iris and Michael (her husband) who is very ill with his legs. They adopted Sean. A wonderful family.

Friday August 11, Dolphin Square

Brother Ian and Margaret's ruby wedding anniversary. They are in a guest room here and I am seeing them tomorrow.

Saturday August 12, Dolphin Square

What made me feel very sad was seeing on TV a film called *The*

Yellow Rolls Royce. I've seen it many times but the first time was when Freddie Ludlow and Sheila Nicholson took me to see it. I miss them both very much. Freddie died almost a year ago and was buried on her birthday, September 22. We were very close and it was a great blow to Freddie when Sheila died.
On the happier side, Ian and Margaret were here, and because their guest room was occupied they've been given, at the same rate, a lovely hotel suite which costs three times as much. They are so happy together and it has been lovely seeing them. It's now nearly 4.00pm, and I am going over to their rooms at 6.15 and we are going out for dinner.
9.40pm. Ian and Margaret took me to the *Pomegranate* for dinner. It has been most enjoyable. We had a long talk about the family, Ma, Jack and Maureen.

Sunday August 13, Dolphin Square

Sylvia telephoned to say that Helen's (Gates) father died; Nettie telephoned to say Norman Gleek died. It's been very close. I didn't swim for long as the pool was crowded. Eddie Davis rang and we had a long chat; Bobby rang and another long chat. I felt tired today because, I think, of the heat, but I feel better this evening. I'm revising - pruning heavily ***501 Days*** - then I'll publish the revised version and will start promoting it.

Monday August 14, Dolphin Square

Just come back (5.30pm) from a sitting with Bill for my second portrait.
Had a letter from Andrew (C) to say he'll be in GOSH tomorrow, and again in September. I'll go in to see him in September as I really ought to work tomorrow. I've got some games for him which Rachel, John Lewis Assistant Toy Buyer, gave me.
Eddie is coming here Saturday to sort out my computer. I'm looking forward to seeing him.

Tuesday August 15, Dolphin Square

Bryan Smith rang to say my Wivenhoe house has been let from October 1st which is good news.
I had a lovely letter, and very touching, from Sam, Nicky's Mum. It seems the Doctors haven't yet finally agreed how much of Nicky's leg has to be amputated, but it looks as if it will be above the knee.

A Russian submarine has sunk in 500 feet of water. The Russians won't let the British and Americans help with the operation to get the men out alive, and it's touch and go whether they will be rescued. Terrible.

Wednesday August 16, Dolphin Square

Had an awful night last night. I couldn't get to sleep. It might have been because I ate two lots of dressed crab Anthea gave me. I hope I have a better night tonight.

Thursday August 17, GOSH

I got a sort of shock today when Maureen (Sister in Alexandra) told me that A.J. unexpectedly had his heart and lung transplant. Maureen said his parents had asked for me so I went to the transplant room in DJW and saw A.J. through the window. He was lying asleep, not to be disturbed, so I stayed for a minute and came away. A.J.'s own heart has gone to another child.

In Parrot I saw, for the first time, Sebastian (Y) aged 4. When he was in the womb something hadn't switched off and half of his brain flooded with blood and had to be removed, leaving him with only 20% sight. He can't talk or walk. He was lying near the window, his father (a Dentist), stroking him gently which comforts the little boy. His father showed great courage and, in the face of this awful tragedy, is hopeful Sebastian will improve, even if it's in a limited way. Two young Physiotherapists came in, put a rug over the floor, and gave Sebastian exercises so I left, but went back to see him later.

In Parrot also I saw Michael (N), aged 13. I've seen him before and he was back for his third operation on a brain tumour. It could only be partly removed as it's too near the brain for further intrusive surgery, but they did operate again this time although I am not sure what happened. I don't like the sound of it. He is such a nice teenager.

Very sad news. Little Zak (G) died at home. He was a lovely child and his Dad said he always liked seeing me. He was 5. He lost his battle with leukaemia. Poor little chap. I wrote to Lorraine and Martin.

Caly is back in Victoria Ward, Chelsea in Alexandra and Jimmy (W) in Clarence. Also Sophia (El-K) is back in Clarence. She was in pain as she's had an operation on her spine. I saw a lot of other children. Going in all day works well as it gives me much more time.

Friday August 18, Dolphin Square

This morning I had a letter from Tracey (J), William's Mum. Also cards from Kay and Keith Jones (Christopher's Uncle and Aunt). And a card from Geraldine, she's in Ireland in her house there.
A large part of this afternoon I spent with Ronnie Page, the Sports Centre manager here. Ronnie and I have been friends for many years and he does a lot for GOSH. He is happily married to Dianne with two lovely children, Katie and William. Hayley (GOSH) sent a most lovely photo of some of the children together with a card to Ronnie to thank him for all he's done for the hospital. The photo and card are now framed and stand either side of the collection box at reception.

Saturday August 19, Dolphin Square

Went to Chelsea today. We beat West Ham 4-2. I went mostly to get programmes for Ben and Tony (A). Tony was in Clarence Ward and is a West Ham supporter. Ben is Chelsea. It's been a lovely sunny, warm afternoon.
This evening I had a long chat to Rosie. I always enjoy chatting to her.
On TV last night was a woman who will eventually be Duchess of Bedford. She was on about people like her being slung out of the House of Lords by Tony Blair; she said it stopped them giving back to the country their privileged education which they'd had the time to be given.

Sunday August 20, Dolphin Square

8.15pm. Martin (Zak's father) has just telephoned. It's very sad. He said Zak, who would have been five years old in two weeks, died suddenly. Martin said it was 5.30am last Wednesday, and as he knew Zak was going he told the little boy he was going to be with the fairies. Zak smiled and died.
This morning and afternoon I felt very, very low and tired. I felt sort of weepy. I wonder if dealing all the time with very ill children, and losing some of them, has an effect on me? I just don't know. Martin said Zak's funeral is next Wednesday but I don't want to go. I find it very upsetting to see the tiny white coffin. I don't like funerals anyway. But I'll write to them nearer the time.

Monday August 21, Dolphin Square

I felt rock-bottom yesterday but today I feel a lot better. I spoke to Stuart in the pool this morning and told him how I felt, and that I thought it might be a culmination of depression in dealing with so many sick children, some of whom have died. Stuart agreed and said that in a different way he sometimes feels down when he gets a very abusive letter (he's high up in the Prosecution Service). He'd had one recently from a very respectable solicitor. He also told me that a top woman barrister had hanged herself because of this. I remember him telling me she had committed suicide but I didn't know why until now.

I had another sitting for my portrait and it's coming on well.

Had a card from Doll Chick thanking me for the flowers I sent for Alby. I'll go and see her soon.

Tuesday August 22, Dolphin Square

Bill introduced me to his son Marcus, a very successful sculptor. Also Marcus' wife Rowena and their baby daughter Theodore. Marcus won first prize in Tokyo for his sculpture there. We had coffee together in the Dolphin Square sandwich bar. Very pleasant.

In a horrific crash on the A1 between a coach carrying teenage air cadets and two lorries, three cadets, two 18 and one 15, were killed. Others were injured, one seriously. Terrible.

Wednesday August 23, Dolphin Square

Ben rang and said he feels better for his operation. I had a card from James (A) who hasn't been feeling too well, which is worrying as he's had leukaemia and a BMT in Robin (I think). Also a letter from Tracey sending me a lovely photograph of William.

Zak's funeral today. Poor little chap.

Thursday August 24, GOSH

I saw in GOSH today lots of old friends who came back: Daniel (P) in Lion Ward and walking now; Rachel (W) in Clarence and little Christopher (E) in Parrot.

I saw A.J. twice. He is still in bed in the transplant room. I bent over to say goodbye and he put his arm round me. He can hardly move or speak and is covered with wires and tubes and I just know, by this gesture, how he feels for me, as I do for him; and I find this with many children, boys and girls. It is the circumstances, I am sure, that they are very sick children and so a very deep and special relationship is built up with many of them. If it means a lot to them, which it seems to, it means a lot to me.

102

I saw Laura (T) who is out of Intensive Care and others; but the most distressing one was Hayley (R),10, who has a movement disorder. She lay shaking in a jerky way, uncontrollably, from head to foot. Her mother, Martine, said Hayley can't sleep with this, and neither she nor Hayley had had any sleep since 12.00 the previous day. When I went later Hayley had been sedated.

Friday August 25, Inverness Train

1.15pm. I've been standing on a packed King's Cross platform for nearly three hours. The train should have left at 12.00 and this only makes watertight my resolution to do no more travelling, not anywhere. Already there is one chap with a loud voice on his mobile phone - he's just spoken of signing off, I hope he means it. Anyway I'll have to put up with whatever happens but I won't do this again.

8.00pm. The train is very late, we will be nearly three hours late getting into Perth. Because of this there was no restaurant car so we've been getting everything free, wine, sandwiches etc.

I got a four-seater because I didn't want to talk, but the lady sitting next to me did, for a time, then she went back to reading *Harry Potter* (the third volume). She does case work for Parliament and was going to see one of her sons who is a farmer near Stirling. She may be a widow as she hadn't her husband with her. She'll be on the train going back on Monday but I don't want to do this journey again, except she told me there's a first class waiting room at King's Cross, which I didn't know, and which is very comfortable with free coffee. So I'll have to think about it and make my mind up next year.

The Lythe, Blairgowrie

11.10pm. I'm too tired to write much. Hugh met me at Perth and we came back to a delicious dinner Brenda had prepared. A hot pot. On the way back in the car Hugh came out with a remark I found quite interesting. He said: *People say you should love God, but how can you love someone you've never met?*

Saturday August 26, The Lythe, Blairgowrie

There hasn't been much to do, but being here is most enjoyable. Quiet, peaceful, lovely surroundings. This morning Brenda, Hugh and I went into Blairgowrie. I bought picture cards of the place and wrote thirteen, quite a few to GOSH children including A.J. and Ben and baby William (J).

Brenda cooked a delicious dinner. A good wine, and liqueur with our coffee in the drawing room afterwards. A most enjoyable day. Now I'm going to bed (11.24pm). Hugh had told me a lot about Lorraine and Geordie I didn't know before, also about Lionel and Sally. I'm too tired tonight so will write about it tomorrow.

Sunday August 27, The Lythe, Blairgowrie

This business with Lorraine and Geordie, and Lionel and Sally, is quite complicated although no more than it has always been. But I think I'll write about it in the train tomorrow as I'll have more time.

It's been a good day. We went to church this morning to *St Ninians*, Alyth. I went there before when I stayed here. This afternoon we went into Blairgowrie. There was Country & Western Music in the Square, followed by the Blairgowrie Pipe Band which was lovely. Girls between 8 - 15 performed Scottish dancing; then the Sailor's Hornpipe by two girls dressed as sailors, then more dancing and country music, but as the band was playing the heavens' opened and it poured. Brenda, Hugh and I got soaked, so we came back and got out of our wet clothes. I enjoyed very much what I saw. This evening we are going out for dinner to the restaurant we went to before, when I last stayed.

Brenda has given me a very nice mobile phone which she didn't want, as her children gave her a small but more expensive one for her handbag.

I've been thinking of A.J. all day. I hope he pulls through.

10.23pm. Just going to bed. We had a super meal at the restaurant called *Lochside*. Very, very nice.

Monday August 28, The Lythe, Blairgowrie

6.35am. I got up early as I'm leaving today. It has been a most enjoyable stay. The dinner, last night, was delicious. I met Jackie again who, I think, owns the restaurant. Her husband is the chef, so Brenda said, and an excellent one. Brenda and I had chump (or rump - I'm not sure) chops, Hugh had chicken. On the way it poured with rain and Hugh had to drive carefully through a couple of deep water troughs that had built up on the side road we travelled along.

Getting back to what Brenda told me about the complications in the Walker-Munro family, these are that the money is not what it was, having been divided out, but they are still an extremely wealthy family. Until he divided it out between Euan and

Geordie, Hugh owned a prosperous farm and a lot of land here, he also has a lot of money. Many years ago one of their legal advisers told me (and this was when their mother was still alive) that each of the four Walker-Munro boys was a millionaire.

Euan, the elder son, is a great success story. He is married to a delightful upper-class girl who herself comes from a wealthy family. They have a daughter, Sophie, and another baby is expected. Euan, when younger joined the Royal Marines as an ordinary Marine and rose to the rank of Lieutenant. He left the Marines, went in for commercial flying, flew helicopters and is now flying jets to Europe and back. He is tall, handsome, charming. Susie, his wife, is very attractive.

Geordie, the second son, and my Godson, is married to Lorraine, who worked in a local video shop. They have two sets of twins. Hugh built a lovely house for them, near his own home, Kinnettles, and then extended the house. I think the cost was about £200,000. He also gave them £40,000 towards their children's education and he made over a substantial amount of land to Geordie which itself brings in an annual income of about £25,000 a year. It has now just gone 7.00am so I'll finish this in the train.

In the train

I've been talking on Perth platform to a very nice person called (Mrs) Sheila Watford. Her father was a test pilot killed in WW2, when his aeroplane caught fire.

In the train - we've just left Perth - I've been told there's a landslide at Berwick and we will probably be very, very late into King's Cross. Just announced there will be severe delays because of the landslide.

Brenda and I also discussed Sally and Lionel. I think she is older than him, but he would be lost without her. But she may outlive him, who can tell.

11.05am. Just been announced that the train is terminating at Edinburgh where we get another train to Dunbar, then a coach to Berwick, then a train from Berwick to King's Cross.

Dolphin Square

10.35pm. I had a very bad journey back although enjoyable and interesting. Will explain tomorrow as I'm too tired to do so tonight. Message on my answering machine from Andy to say Gemma has had a baby boy called Hayden.

Tuesday August 29, Dolphin Square

Yesterday I left Perth on the 9.56am. We were told there was a landslide at Berwick and our train would terminate at Edinburgh, which it did. Almost unbelievably, the same person who had sat next to me going to Perth had the same seat booked next to me going back.

When we got to Edinburgh we stood around for over an hour, no-one telling us anything. Then we demanded from an official that he sort something out, and he got permission for us to go on a Virgin train to Carlisle and change there for London. At Edinburgh I met a very nice young man, William Wu, aged 23, high up in the computer world. He and I went together on the Virgin train, while the lady who had sat next to me went to look for a first-class seat. I didn't bother with this as I knew all the carriages were full and there weren't any seats anywhere.

On the way to Carlisle more people got in and the train was packed, which reminded me of seeing the crowded trains taking Jewish men, women and children to Auschwitz. As a matter of fact a lot of orthodox Jews, men, women and small children got into our train at Carlisle, adding to the crowd there.

At Carlisle we changed to the London train. I went with William and we had to stand packed together in the corridor of a standard compartment, all (with the exception of me of course) young people. We were so full there was not even room to sit on the floor.

One young man near me, like William, was a computer expert from South Africa, another an engineer while another worked for Sony on the technical side of music. He and William talked at high level on various technical matters. There was also a young very attractive New Zealand social worker, and a young Australian and his wife - she was doing research and experiments with blood (I think in Oxford). There were also two Japanese girl students studying English at a University (Tokyo I think). They were lovely; both had caught the wrong train, ending up in London instead of Lancaster. One is called Kaoru, the other Kei.

At Euston (we arrived there instead of King's Cross because of changing onto Virgin) William and I sorted out the Japanese girls. We bought them coffee and sandwiches and put them on the right train, in charge of the Guard, for Lancaster. And this is the strange thing, I very much enjoyed the journey back with those youngsters even though I'd had to stand squashed up for seven hours. Much better than having to listen to boring conversations of first-class passengers.

Wednesday August 30,Dolphin Square

I've made a list of priority work which I want to finish as quickly as possible. The most important is to get out all my diaries; these will finish altogether in the year 2000. There are ten volumes. Then I want to get out the revised version of *501 Days*. After this I hope to start on *Vision of Glory,* the fourth Forsyth book. Plenty to do.

Thursday August 31, GOSH

A.J. is greatly improved. He was out in a wheelchair twice. He speaks quietly and hoarsely but has still some way to go.
In Fox I saw Natasha, unfortunately her leukaemia has returned. I also saw Ismael, Stanley and Jack. In Clarence I saw Samuel, Michael (S) an only child, Sophia (El-K), and Ricky. Kev from Barnardo's is with Ricky all the time. I'm not sure of Ricky's age. He looks about 12, but can't communicate. He has beautiful brown eyes but lies staring into space, sometimes following a movement with his eyes, the serious expression on his face fixed. His hands are doubled up all the time. Kev is devoted to him, which speaks volumes for Barnardo's who are very caring.
Charlotte (J), who is in a wheelchair when she is not in bed, was in Alexandra with her mother. She is very handicapped but always laughing. I've known her a long time.
Aleema, in Transitional Care, had deteriorated; she was making good progress, then had respiratory problems and went into Intensive Care. Now she has improved. She can't talk properly but moves her mouth. She is a beautiful girl with a devoted mother.
Emma was in Fox / Robin reception. The last time I saw her she had been ill with food poisoning. She said she was very sick but is now better.
I ended up in Victoria Ward with Lucy (M) who is (I think) 14. She's a lovely girl and was there with her mother Angela. Lucy is waiting for a kidney transplant when one becomes available.

Friday September 1, Dolphin Square

Today I wrote to ten American University Law Schools. Loren Geistfeld had very kindly sent me the names and addresses. It was very good of him as he is extremely busy with his own work.

Peter Holloway rang to say the proof of Volume Four of my diary will be delivered on Monday morning; so that will be quite a big job as I have to go through it, also get out a numbered index.

Saturday September 2, Dolphin Square

Spent today with Andy, Jane, Gemma and baby Hayden who is a week old. He is a beautiful baby. So good.

Sunday September 3, Dolphin Square

I telephoned Jane to say I've booked a table for the 21st at the R M-S. I enjoyed the day with them yesterday. The only black mark is Andy's smoking. He won't give it up. He's crazy to continue but I'm sick of telling him. He's been banned from smoking indoors now that Hayden has arrived; he should have been banned a long time ago. Ali, Anita and the children have been there today.

This evening I watched some of Steven Spielberg's *E.T. The Extra-Terrestial*. A brilliant film, a modern classic. The ending is so moving with the human boy and the Alien, their arms around each other, saying goodbye. It says it all about the sadness of parting for ever, and I thought of one of the saddest sights I ever saw in GOSH, when Christopher's Mother was bending over her dying son, and he reached up and clasped her, and they were like this for some time. Not long after, Christopher, 15, died in PICU.

Monday September 4, Dolphin Square

Iris, Sean's mother, telephoned to say Ben (G), who went to the school for handicapped children where Sean goes, had died aged 6. Iris thought I knew Ben, but it was Zak (G) I knew at GOSH. The proof for Volume Four of my diaries came today. I also had another sitting for my portrait with Bill. He fixed up my mobile for me, which is now working.

Tuesday September 5, Dolphin Square

I've had another busy day. Had letters from Emma (U) and Shabnam and a card from France from Byron. I get quite a lot of letters and cards from GOSH children, which is very nice.

The Twins' (Lionel and Hugh) birthday. But Lionel I don't see at all now. I've had an introduction from the New Zealand High Commission to five New Zealand universities (law libraries) for **The Trial**, so have written to all five.

Wednesday September 6, Dolphin Square

A letter today from the Fitzmaurices whom I met in GOSH when Scott was there.

I've had a good day, working mostly on the index for Volume Four of the diaries. Redwood books are excellent. Peter Holloway, who looks after everything to do with me is very efficient, and very nice.

Am leaving shortly (it's now nearly 4.30pm) to meet Ali at Earl's Court for the Chelsea v Arsenal match at Stamford Bridge.

Thursday September 7, GOSH

I saw A.J. briefly. He's out a lot more, and leaving Tuesday for a hospice. He's making good progress.

I met little Ellie (H), aged 5, in Clarence. She's so bright and cheerful and has a rare disease that weakens the bones in her legs, so that she wobbles when she walks or runs. She's gorgeous.

I also saw Danny (P), aged 5, in Helena. He's very bright too, a lovely little boy. Sophia was in bed in Clarence, she's better but still in a bit of pain. Next to her is Ricky - I've written about him before. He just stares with a fixed expression, but his Mum told me he gets to all the Arsenal home matches and sometimes goes abroad to football matches. Amazing, the courage of these parents, and their children.

In Parrot I saw Kerry (W) ,15, who had miraculously survived being knocked down by a motor-bike and falling on her head. Also little Sahil (A), a pretty dark 5-year-old. She can't speak English but her Dad can a little, also her Mum who, too, is lovely.

Peter (L) who runs the GOSH Radio Station told me about Prince Philip's visit there. Peter said that when he was asked to sign the visitors' book, Prince Philip said he didn't give autographs. Maybe Peter's got it muddled. Saw Andy (S). I like him. He supervises Security.

Friday September 8, Dolphin Square

Priority is getting out my page-numbered index for Volume Four of the diaries. But I want to do, even a little, of **Vision of Glory**. It's fun getting exactly the right words.

I wish Frank Jackson was still here.

Saturday September 9, Dolphin Square

Most of today I'v been working on the index for Volume Four of the diaries.

Sunday September 10, Dolphin Square

I am pruning *501 Days* to make it more commercially acceptable. But the priority is the index to Volume Four of the diaries.

Yesterday (or the day before) Muriel Spark was on TV. It's funny how every successful author is the greatest English writer living. There are quite a few of them. But she is very successful, and writes well, and interestingly. She is now on another book and researching material for it. You just have to go on as best you can and for as long as you can.

Monday September 11, Dolphin Square

I keep Monday afternoons free for Bill who is working on the second portrait of me. He is very good, and I like the portraits. He said this afternoon, in so many words, that you can't tell what may happen in the future in terms of commercial success.

I've been working on the index for a good part of today.

Tuesday September 12, Dolphin Square

David, from the carpenter's shop, came in to measure two shelves for my kitchen. I had written to Miriam in Maintenance and she very kindly arranged it for me, as the carpenters are always busy. This afternoon I went to see Dr Corbett-B. I'm not sure what the B stands for. She is so nice. I like lady doctors. She took my blood pressure and tested my heart and said I am OK. She said she has two teenage children. I think one is at Eton.

Had two very nice thank-you letters from Barry and Karl (Stapleton). Geraldine went through so much when Barry was in GOSH with leukaemia and cancer behind the eye. I hope, more than anything, he stays in remission.

Wednesday September 13, Dolphin Square

I had an email from the University of Virginia asking for a copy of *The Trial* which I have sent; and I had a letter from Ellen Bannach who has just got a new job in her local German University Library (she lives in Jena). She said some of my books, two of the Forsyth books and some of the diaries, are listed there. That's really good.

Thursday September 14, GOSH

A.J. is looking much better. He's back for a check-up as his new lungs weren't 100%, but I gather this is not unusual in a lung transplant, and he's had lung and heart. A girl, who also had a lung and heart transplant, has just been rushed back and is very ill. I hope she has survived. I haven't heard to the contrary. I saw Ricky in Clarence. A Carer from Barnardo's was with him, also his mother. He was supposed to be going to theatre but this was postponed until tomorrow. He just lies there, more or less expressionless, his hands curled under his arms, bent. His eyes (beautiful eyes) move towards you. I am certain there is some communication.

I couldn't see any of my little friends in Fox Ward as there is a chicken pox scare and they were all (fed up with having to do it) in their rooms with red labels on the doors.

In Victoria I saw Nickesh (K), 15. I think he had had a kidney transplant and is making good progress. I also saw Laura (T) who was in a wheelchair by the volunteers' desk in the reception area. She looked much, much better. I was going back to see her in DJW before I went, but I didn't; but when I saw her I gave her money for sweets.

In Parrot I found Mark (E) who had come back because he was getting headaches, and had sharp pains in both his legs. At the time I saw him the doctors hadn't diagnosed what was wrong. Hopefully it is nothing serious. He is tall, good-looking and has his mother's features. I told him if he'd gone home by the time I was in again I would post him his favourite sweets - wine gums, those I get from Marks.

In Parrot also I saw William Harkness. We had a chat. He is now one of the world's leading neuro-surgeons. He obtained permission from the Sister to allow me into the operating theatre for the day, where I saw him carry out two brain operations; in the morning removing a large brain tumour from a little 4-year-old Greek girl, and in the afternoon performing a leucotomy on a 10-year-old boy, where the brain is snipped to prevent fits. With the little girl, when the top of the skull was removed, William let me look inside, and it was so beautiful, white and scarlet.

Friday September 15, Dolphin Square

In the launderette this afternoon I met Alix, a French doctor who practises here. She wants a copy of my diary. While I was in the launderette the power failed. The whole of Dolphin Square was without electricity. Nothing working, only my battery wireless which I put on for the 5.00pm news. I've never known such a complete breakdown in all the fifty years I've lived here. I had to walk up nine flights of stairs as the lifts weren't working, which

I managed OK. The breakdown continued until very late - nearly midnight. It just shows how dependent modern society is on man-made conveniences. My electric clock wasn't working, nor my lighting, nor my answering machine - nothing that depends on electricity, only my little clocks and wireless, that work on batteries.

Saturday September 16, Dolphin Square

I've had an excellent day. Eddie came here this morning and stayed until 5.00pm. The day passed so quickly. Eddie tried to put *words* on my computer instead of *works*. He nearly got there, but he didn't want to risk my having nothing, so he's left it until he gets a *works* disc otherwise I might be left with nothing.

Sunday September 17, Dolphin Square

Battle of Britain Day - 60th anniversary. My thoughts are with Bill Lundon, but they always are, regardless of anniversaries. I was particularly interested in what one woman, who took part in the TV programme on the Battle, said. At the time she was eight years old and saw a young British pilot, who had been shot down, descending in his parachute. As he came down a German Messersmit circled the pilot and machine gunned him as he descended.
An ARP Warden went over, came back and said to the little girl: *He's torn to ribbons.* She said (now in old age): *I've never ever forgotten those words, and from that moment I saw the reality and horror of war* (these may not be the exact words, but near enough). They moved me very much.
Went to Chelsea, principally to get a programme for Ben. Chelsea lost to Leicester 2.0.

Monday September 18, Dolphin Square

It's been an interesting day, rather bitty, although I've got quite a lot of things done. This evening Eddie rang me from his home in Cambridge; he connected up his computer to mine so that we could communicate on computer problems. He is a very kind person and a good friend.

Tuesday September 19, Dolphin Square

It's been a bitty day today as well. As well as my usual weekly visit to M & S foods (Pantheon) I went to Peter Jones and bought among other things some quite expensive ink. The girl said it's the best and it's £5 a pot instead of £3.45 (Quink). It's called Mont Blanc and cleans as it writes or something like this, but I haven't used it much as I've got quite a few bottles of Quink left. I do think, with reliable brands, you get what you pay for.

Thursday September 21, Dolphin Square

I took Andy and Jane to the Mid-Surrey for dinner. We had a very pleasant evening. Ted and Glen Bennett were there. Had a chat with them.

Friday September 22, GOSH

Freddie's birthday. Her funeral took place on her birthday last year.

This evening a nurse in Parrot Ward told me that my ward visiting means a lot to the hospital. She really did sing my praises, which was very flattering, but although it was very nice of her and heart-warming; all that matters to me are the children and their parents whom I see and get to know.

I had a letter from Sue (S), Anna's Mum. To quote some of it: *As we live quite a way from London, and couldn't have many visitors, it was really nice to see you every Thursday. It's not just the children who appreciate your visits but the mums too!....... Thank you very much again. You are greatly appreciated - Sue S.*

Anna also sent me a card and a lovely photograph of herself.

The day before I had a letter from Edward's (Geffen) Mum, Camilla, asking me if I would write to Edward at the Dragon School in Oxford, where he has just started. Edward, who is 8, had a brain tumour removed when he was 5. He is a delightful boy, and of course I have written to him.

I went into GOSH today instead of Thursday to see Andrew (G-C),15, as I had some crossword games for him which Rachel had given me. Andrew looked a lot better than when I saw him in Clarence, where he had a spinal fusion.

I also saw Matthew (T) whose leg is still in a cage and who was in for a day clinic. He looked bright and cheerful as usual.

Patrick (B), 4, was still in Annie Zunz Ward. Andy (Security) gave me A.J.'s telephone number which A.J. had asked him to give me. I saw Kevin (N) who was having a check-up in Elephant Day Care; a very nice boy from Doncaster who is in remission from leukaemia. I could go on writing about all my little friends, but I must mention Abdul (A) and Nathan (B-W) who were in Alexandra for their check-ups. Abdul said we have known each other for two years, and it must be at least a year I've known Nathan.

Sister Maureen told me A.J. would have died if he hadn't had the heart and lung transplant, because although his heart was OK his lungs were almost destroyed by disease. Maureen told me also that Ben is OK because his lungs aren't too bad; it's his lower region, bowels etc., where it's gone wrong. But it's not life-threatening. I was relieved to hear this. She said Ben won't be coming back to GOSH.

Saturday September 23, Dolphin Square

Chelsea drew with Manchester United away, which was good news. We have a new manager.

Sunday September 24, Dolphin Square

Alistair Perriam and I correspond a lot by email (he's in Spain). He has a delightful personality.

Monday September 25, Dolphin Square

Had an email from Ellen Bannach in Jena, asking me to send copies of **Violence, The Trial** and two diaries recently published, for the University library.

On the TV news it showed an Australian bay where a teenager and another man had gone surfing and had been killed (presumably eaten since their bodies haven't been found) by white sharks. It seemed crazy to me they should have gone surfing when they must have known the danger, but I couldn't help thinking that there are always people worse off.

Tuesday September 26, Dolphin Square

An order came today, to Destination Way, for the first three of the Forsyth books from an Eastbourne bookshop. It had come through Whitakers. As I don't do any marketing it just shows what can happen. I felt the same pleasure that I got when the trainee barrister wrote to say he'd found **The Trial** in Lincoln's Inn library, and wanted to buy a copy for himself.

Wednesday September 27, Dolphin Square

Had a most interesting letter from Byron today, telling me about his school, his holidays and so on, and that he's coming to GOSH in March.

Thursday September 28, GOSH

I've said before that to see a dying child is the saddest of all situations. I went to Lion Ward to see Alfie (S) who is 8. I've known him for some time, and when they X-rayed him recently, to have a possible operation, they found the tumour had spread everywhere and nothing can be done. He is very pale and thin, and was going back home this afternoon. He is a lovely child. I gave him some money to buy sweets and he just said: *Thank you William.* I don't think he's got long to go, and of course his parents, Debbie and Roy, who are with him all the time, know the situation. It is so awful for them.

Then I saw little Lily (B), aged 4, who has neuroblastoma stage IV. This is what Sue, her Mum, wrote in my book. I don't know what it means, not being a doctor, but I imagine it's a severe form of leukaemia, as Lily is in Fox Ward. I'll find out when I'm there next time. I'll ask Maggie, the Sister, if she's on duty.

I also saw Laura (M), 6, who was in Alexandra Ward; she should have been in Dickens but there wasn't a bed available. Caroline, Laura's Mum, told me the local hospital diagnosed Laura incorrectly as having arthritis, and this went on for two months until she came to GOSH. She has a narrowing of the oesophagus. Caroline told me she lost her son Stephen, aged four months, in 1955. I've said it before and I'll say it again, that so often the courage of parents I deal with in GOSH is beyond belief.

In Alice I met Lik-Mun, a beautiful young nurse. I met her when the two of us came to GOSH five years ago, and sat together in Occupational Health, where you went for a health examination when you first joined GOSH. How time flies.

Abdul was still in Alexandra, so was Nathan but he was at school. Little Yasmin was asleep.

I met a delightful Greek Cypriot boy, Erodotos, aged 11. He has quite a lot wrong with him and is in Nuffield Ward (Private Patients). You can easily run up £100,000 so most children in the Nuffield Wards are paid for by their governments, and the money helps GOSH.

In the evening, at 5.00pm, I collected Ingibjörg from the Italian Hospital where she had been on reception. We went on to the Mid-Surrey Golf Club for dinner. Barry, her husband, is in Australia. We had a lovely evening. Inga is marvellous company. On Waterloo Station we bumped into Ros (GOSH). Fortunately the weather stayed dry and sunny.

Friday September 29, Dolphin Square

I've been working on the index for Volume Four today.
I sent a card with £5 for Alfie. I see he has neuroblastoma, the same as Lily.

Saturday September 30, Dolphin Square

Just got back from a visit to Martyn and Pauline. I took them to lunch at the Black Buoy (Wivenhoe); then on to John and Isobel where I had an early supper. I took some flowers to the cemetery for Edwin.

When I got back I found a message on my answering machine from Iris to say Sean died yesterday at 5.00pm. Sean has been ill all his short life with fits and other problems. He's had a lot wrong. Most of the time I saw him, he was lying back in his special chair, his eyes closed.

He had so much love and care from Iris and Michael, who adopted him, and from their family and friends. The message from Iris was simple:

Hullo, William, it's Iris. I spoke to you yesterday to tell you Sean was very, very poorly. I'm afraid that he died yesterday evening. I'll speak to you during the week sometime and have a little chat about it. Bye.

Sunday October 1, Dolphin Square

I went to Chelsea for the first half. I came away then because I don't like crowds. We beat Liverpool 3-0. I bought Ben a programme. It was enjoyable - sunny and warm. Betty rang and we had a long chat.

Michael Walker-Munro's birthday.

Monday October 2, Dolphin Square

Most of today I've been working on the index to Volume Four.

Tuesday October 3, Dolphin Square

Alan Neame telephoned this afternoon. I haven't heard from him for ages, so I was glad to hear his voice. We are very old and close friends and he's helped me in many ways, especially with writing.

5.10pm. I've been working again on the index to Volume Four of the diaries. I had a newsy letter from Carol (F) about Scott and the family.

Wednesday October 4, Dolphin Square

New York University came in today for two Forsyth books (email): *Violence* and *The Trial.* I had told them about *The Trial* but they found *Violence* in their bibliographical records. My books are building up gradually.

Gemma sent me a lovely photograph of little Hayden.

Ordinary letters have more or less finished, but I get a lot of letters and cards from GOSH children, and sometimes parents. I love corresponding with them and it helps them. They are beautiful children and bear so bravely so much suffering and (especially their parents) anxiety.

This evening we start French classes under Anne (Rivoire). She is a super teacher.

Thursday October 5, Dolphin Square

I'm very pleased with the acceptance of *The Trial* by the American Universities. I had the University of Chicago in today, and New York yesterday. They were also interested in Volume 1, *Violence*.

Had a letter from Rhoda who very kindly said she will proof read the index for Volume Four of my diaries which I should finish this weekend.

Friday October 6, GOSH

Went into GOSH today specially to see Scott (R). Janice and Steve (Scott's Carer) were there, in Clarence. Scott smiled at some of what I said to him. He lies back in his chair and it could be, for those who don't know him well, he might not appear to be taking in what is said. He has grown a lot and is a handsome youngster. I was told he got brain damage as a baby when he fell into a shallow pond. A great tragedy, but he has so much love and care, which all the children at GOSH have from their families, and nurses and doctors. It's one of the marvellous things about working at GOSH, you see the best of human nature there. Among the sick children, very sick children, you see the very best of what human beings mean to each other in terms of help, support and comfort, and unselfishness.

This morning I had a letter from Sam enclosing a painting from Nicholas. Sam is expecting her third child in three weeks. I'll write to Nicky soon. He's got to come into GOSH to get his leg sorted out. It may have to be amputated.

Went up to Nuffield Ward to see Erodotos. He is Cypriot, a delightful boy aged 11. He is having tests. Today is his birthday. I left a card and chocolate for him as he was at school. I intended going back to see him, but didn't have time as I am going out to see the Stapletons.

I had a wonderful evening. Geraldine cooked the most delicious meal. All the family were there, Kevin, Kieran, Danielle, Barry and Karl.

Saturday October 7, Dolphin Square

I've been working all day on my pamphlet. I had intended finishing the index for Volume Four of the diaries but Bill came in at 10.15am, and said it is urgent I get out the pamphlet on my books and diaries, so I sat all day until 6.30pm, and finished it. Bill then made some alterations and it is now ready to send out. I'll start with New York and Chicago on Monday.

This evening I watched a TV programme on the opening of the Second World War. An officer (now retired) said that when the German dive-bombers were bombing fleeing civilians one of his soldiers was blown off his bike and found himself beside a little boy whose legs had been blown off and had lost the sight of an eye. The soldier took the child in his arms, saw he was dying and in great pain, so took his revolver and shot the child. Later he asked his officer (Peter Vaux) if he had done the right thing. The officer said he had done the right thing, and he would have done the same. Isn't war dreadful?

Sunday October 8, Dolphin Square

I'm going to write to Peter Vaux and see if he will tell me more about that poor child whose legs were blown off by the German bomber pilot. It is the pilot, not the bomber; it is the man blowing up women and children. Totally evil. There were brave Germans (like Bonhoeffer) but as a nation, certainly then, they were an evil lot. Strange that *both* my grandmothers were German. Also the Consultant at Chelsea & Westminster Hospital, who examined me for my last annual check-up, a very caring person, was German.

Monday October 9, Dolphin Square

As I have said, I get lovely letters from children and parents. I had an email from Margaret (H) today, and the PS said: *All these Olympians received medals for their great achievements. I think*

*you should, too, for the happiness you bring to kids - I wish you
could have seen D's (David) face when he received your postcard.*
I don't look for praise or thanks, but it is a warming to know you
are helping children in this way.

Last night on TV there was a very realistic play - obviously
auto-biographical - about a child sexually abused by one of the
staff, a fat middle-aged man; and it gave the history of children
in these homes who have suffered unspeakable abuse and
torment. Terrible.

7.30pm. Richard Green, a friend (or relation?) of the Geffen
family, has just telephoned with the very sad news that Edward,
aged 8, died suddenly. I saw a lot of Edward at GOSH, and when
he came for a check-up he always left me a note. I've got many of
these now. He was a handsome boy. Very, very sad. I feel so sorry
for his parents, Robin and Camilla.

9.00pm. I feel so sad over Edward, but I have to face up to it that
if I work with very sick children it is inevitable some won't make
it. I get so fond of them, it's as bad as losing one of my own. In a
way, they are mine.

This evening I wrote this letter to Peter Vaux c/o Peter Craig,
Producer, Book-Lapping Productions:

*I watched with great interest Finest Hour on BBC 2 on
Saturday. I am nearly 82 and was in the Navy during the war,
but I still research into all aspects of war, especially the more
personal side. For example, in this programme, one of our
soldiers shot a German soldier, but thought of the German's
family and whispered to himself The Lord's Prayer, which I
found very moving.*

*But what I found even more moving was the account you gave of
the soldier who found himself alongside a child of five, whose legs
had been blown off by German bombing, who was half blind and
dying, and the soldier shot the child to put the little boy out of his
pain, then later said to you: Did I do the right thing sir?, and you
said yes, I would have done it myself.*

*The brutality of war is a little softened by these acts of great
compassion, because it must have been the most difficult thing to
do, to kill a child for whatever reason. I have such admiration for
that soldier.*

*I didn't get quite clear whether he was an officer. He called you sir,
and could have been a junior officer. He used a revolver which I
thought only officers carried. If I am not troubling you too much
could you tell me more about him, if he is still alive and what his*

rank was? It would be nice to know his name if you are able to say, but I would understand if you can't. But I would just like to know more about him and the incident.

It was a beautifully produced programme, with such clear commentary throughout. It also brought back memories. I saw Churchill close up several times.

Tuesday October 10, Dolphin Square

THE TIMES, TUESDAY OCTOBER 10, 2000

GEFFEN - *Edward Robin Henry, aged 8 while on exeat from the Dragon School, Oxford, suddenly but peacefully on October 3rd 2000 in Southampton Central Hospital. Deeply adored eldest son of Camilla and Robin, beloved brother and best friend of William, also dearly loved grandson of Martin and Anthea Busk and Maureen and Henry Buckley. His boundless enthusiam for everything and steadfast courage will always be an inspiration to us. A special boy whose huge smile warmed all who knew him. Funeral Service at All Saints Church, Houghton, near Stockbridge, Hampshire on Thursday 12th October at 3pm. Family flowers only, but donations to Great Ormond Street Children's Hospital may be sent to A H Chester, Funeral Directors, 122 The Hundred, Romsey, Hampshire, SO51 8BY.*

Wednesday October 11, GOSH

Edward's unexpected death is very, very sad. He always left me little notes in my in-tray, when in GOSH, which I've kept. I'll miss him. I miss every child I've lost.

Saw Erodotos (M) in Nuffield. He is having a major operation on Monday. I think he's having one kidney removed, but Professor Spitz will cut him all round his right side, a long cut so that he can have a thorough look inside to see what is causing other problems. Erodotos is a charming youngster and, like all the children and their parents, very courageous.

Emma (T) is back in Alice. She is now 15, has osteophenia and Dystrophic Epidermdysia Bullose (this is what her Mum wrote in my notebook). She has bad, very bad skin and her bones are bad so that she is in constant pain, and has continuous morphine, but she is chatty and smiling. A lovely girl. So is Sophia (El-K) who was back in Clarence, also in pain with spinal problems. She and Emma are close friends, and she said they are hoping to meet for lunch tomorrow.

I took a pot of purple heather to the chapel for Edward. Noel and Jill came out, and Jill walked along with me. I spoke about the loss of a child, and Jill, who is GOSH assistant Chaplain, told me that she had lost her little son, David, aged 5, twenty-two years ago. She said she had felt angry and asked God why he had done this but then, after a time, although her life changed completely and was never the same again, she learned to accept it. She has two daughters, both married, one with an adopted child. You learn acceptance but the loss never goes away.

I saw Pauric (O). He is over from Ireland for a check-up. I last saw him in August. His Mum had put in my book *virus, Robin.* Robin is the bone marrow transplant ward. Anyhow Pauric looked well so I hope his check-up is OK. He is staying in one of the GOSH flats for a couple of days. Saw June (I) near the volunteer's desk.

I went to two parties: the annual volunteers' party and then on to the party to celebrate the 20th anniversary of Radio GOSH. Both very enjoyable.

Thursday October 12, Dolphin Square

Brother Alan telephoned this evening to say that Wendy's mother died. She was 89. He said after speaking to me he was going to telephone Babs in Canada.

Friday October 13, Dolphin Square

I've been working on the proof of my 1963-65 diary all day. I went down this afternoon to post some letters and bumped into Ronnie Page in our Sports Centre. We sat and talked for three-quarters of an hour. Ronnie likes my diaries and always buys a copy. We have been good friends for many years. I knew him when he was single; he's married to Dianne and has two lovely children, Katie and William. He said he chose William for his son because he knows four Williams he liked including me. I felt flattered. Ronnie does so much for GOSH, sending in collection box after collection box.

Had an email from Janice to say Scott hasn't had the results of his tests, but his Baclofen pump is malfunctioning so he'll have to come in for that.

I've sent an email to Ben as he is in the middle of severe flooding in the Kent and Sussex areas. I couldn't get through on the telephone. Also sent a letter to Sophia who is still in Clarence.

Saturday October 14, GOSH

Went to the annual Transitional Care party in Coram Fields. I saw quite a few of my little friends, Aleema, Matthew, Keelan and many others. The party is run beautifully.

Spoke to Jill Pryor on the telephone. She helped me with a computer problem, then we had a general chat.

Sunday October 15, Dolphin Square

Have had a very busy day. This morning, until 2.30pm I wrote to GOSH parents and children - about nine letters. But, as Sylvia said when I told her, it's no effort as it comes from the heart. Sylvia also told me something I never knew, that when she was ten she lost her eight-year-old sister, Doreen, the twin of her brother Don. Both twins had diphtheria, and although she seemed to be the stronger of the two he got better and Doreen didn't. Sylvia said she still remembers Doreen's smiling face.

Nearly 8.00pm and Alan (brother) telephoned and went on for quite a time, unusual for him. He said when he gets too old for golf etc. he's going to write his history. It's good to be occupied.

I was looking at a letter from Vera, Christopher's Grandmother. She wrote the words he is going to have on his head-stone:

> We lived in hope and prayed in vain
> That God would make you well again.
> He took your hand, we had to part,
> He eased your pain but broke our hearts.

A note left in my in-tray from Annette (M) didn't give very good news about little James. There's nothing more can be done for him. Very worrying.

Monday October 16, Dolphin Square

Went to Peter Jones and bought a combined answering, fax and email machine (Sagem). It was recommended to me by Michael Percival who lives here. He is a talented actor.

I bumped into Salina, or rather she bumped into me. She was in a van with Roy and I had just come out of Peter Jones. A hug and a kiss: it was lovely seeing her again, and him.

Tuesday October 17, Dolphin Square

Yesterday I had this email from the University of Chicago:

I am writing again to let you know that we will be adding the additional volume you sent, The Hanging of Floss Forsyth, Book 1, Violence, to our collection, and that we would also like to receive

Vols 3 & 4 in the Floss Forsyth series when they are available - Sheila Ralston.

Wednesday October 18, Dolphin Square

Been all day finishing the index for Volume Four of the diaries. Rhoda posted the proof-read version. It is so kind of her to do this for me.

Just going to French class. Anne Rivoire takes us. I like her very much.

Thursday October 19, GOSH

I put some white roses in the chapel for Sarah (E) whose anniversary was 12 October.

Bumped into Bashrat (M) who had been in Victoria with kidney problems. He was in for the day and looked well, I was pleased to see.

Sophia was still in Clarence. And in the next bed a lovely little boy called Edward (G), aged 4. He was having a lump under the skin investigated and was being transferred to Alice, which is the skin ward.

In Alexandra I saw Victoria (T),13, who has cystic fibrosis; also little Yasmin who is sweet. She had woken up so I talked to her.

In Nuffield Erodotos was recovering from his major operation. The first time I saw him he was asleep, but in the evening he was up in a wheelchair, quite bright, a courageous boy, and charming. He is a Greek Cypriot.

In Parrot I saw Samantha (W),13, whose brain tumour, unfortunately, had returned, but fortunately had been picked up in the beginning by tests. In the bed opposite was Aleena (K) ,3, who'd had a blood clot on the brain.

Riza (A), whom I first saw in Dialysis, was later downstairs, and she told me it's her 13th birthday on Monday 23rd, so I've sent her a card.

In Dialysis I saw Michael and Freddie: they like sweets called Kinder Surprise.

I met for the first time Steven (G) who was out for the first day after a bone marrow transplant. In Transitional Care I saw Aleema who tries to speak, but her lips shape words, and she can't do more than that, and can't move. I'm not quite sure what is wrong. She is a very sick child, a beautiful face. I've known her for some time now.

In Fox Ward I saw little Lewis (R), nearly 3, who has

Neuroblastoma, not all that rare in the cancer wards, as I've dealt with other children who have it. I think Lily in Fox has it but am not quite sure. I saw her, but I'll find out next time. Bill (P), 4, has had a relapse with Wilms Tumour. Natasha (van H), 18 months, also in Fox, has had a relapse with AML.

Friday October 20, Dolphin Square

Most of today has been taken up with my new Sagem email, fax and answering machine.

Saturday October 21, Dolphin Square

I've had a busy day including getting ready Volume Five of my diaries. There's a lot to do.

Sunday October 22, Dolphin Square

Took Richard and Barbara Doyle-Davidson to the Royal Mid-Surrey Golf Club for lunch. It was a very nice lunch and I enjoyed seeing them. Richard proposed me for the club about forty years ago. I also saw Ted and Glen Bennett, but as I don't go all that often I don't know so many people. I bumped into (brother) Alan who was there, but was leaving just as I saw him.
Eddie rang me this evening and taught me how to use the computer telephone.

Monday October 23, Dolphin Square

Mike Newland drove me to Eltham to see the Stephen Lawrence memorial. It was sad to stand there where he had stood when he was stabbed to death by white thugs. There were flowers on the paving stone that had the inscription.

Tuesday October 24, Dolphin Square

I wrote to Marjorie (Baker) today in reply to a letter she had written to me. In her letter she wrote:
I am going to see Jackie, our grandaughter, who is coming up to her final year at Northampton University doing English Literature. She has always been a great reader like her Grandfather......Whilst I am in Northampton we are going to wander around trying to see where Cyril lived and went to school when he was fostered there. We found out about his life at Barnardo's, things he hadn't remembered, a few days before he went into hospital. A person from Barnardo's came up from London and went through Cyril's file with him and it seemed to give him great satisfaction. So that is how I knew about the house

and the school of which Cyril had happy memories.
I have a lot of time for Barnardo's. In GOSH we have a Barnardo's boy Ricky, in Clarence. A Carer from Barnardo's is with Ricky all the time.
Not long ago on TV they showed a brilliant young violinist who was from Barnardo's, and Barnardo's had paid for her to have special tuition. A wonderful and caring home.

Wednesday October 25, Dolphin Square

When I had a sitting this evening with Bill for my portrait, he said that I had had the most interesting life of anyone he knew. Quite a few people, from time to time, have told me that; so although there have been a lot of difficulties, it's been worth it.

Thursday October 26, Dolphin Square

Rita Mundy and I went to Island Garden (Docklands) to have lunch with Judy and David Longbottom. It has been a lovely sunny day. The lunch, which David cooked, was delicious. Both Rita and I enjoyed it enormously. I should have met up with Rita on the Central Line Bank platform, but I worked out incorrectly which side she would be (my fault) so we missed each other, and when I got to Judy's she was there. But we came back together.
There are all sorts of rumblings at Dolphin Square, that Westminster City Council are trying to break the lease, which means I could lose my low rent. But I'm told they would have to pay compensation, so I'll wait and see.

Friday October 27, GOSH

When I got to GOSH I went to the Italian Hospital as Inga was on duty, and we had a long talk. I am trying to help her get a gallery for her mosaics, which are so beautiful. They are collector's items, very, very lovely.
Inga said that in time my diaries will become popular. She said she wasn't being nice, she meant it. I know she meant it, and although I have such a lack of confidence in anything I do I am sure, in my heart, she is right.
In Lion Ward a Nurse took me on one side to tell me two of the children had died. One of them was Jake. It was good of her to do this, but I had already written to Jake's parents. The other child I didn't know but I thanked her for telling me.
In Parrot Ward I saw Courtney (L), aged 2. She had a fractured skull. Zoe, her Mum, told me Courtney had got out of bed early in the morning, opened the French windows, something that had

125

never happened before, and fell fifteen feet onto the balcony below. Fortunately, although the balcony was concrete, it broke her fall. Had she fallen right to the bottom (it was a tall block of flats) she would almost certainly have been killed. She is in for observation and seems to be recovering.

In Parrot also I saw Molly (P), 10, who is having her shunt seen to; Gemma (R), 12, also having her shunt dealt with; and little Aleema (K), 3, whom I had seen before: she has a blood clot in the brain and can see - but not very well - only black and white. Also in Parrot Samantha (W), 13, who had had a brain tumour.

In PICU I saw George (P), 14 months, who has a chest infection, and Joshua (S), 3, who has respiratory problems.

I saw my little friends in Fox and Robin. They are long-term in these wards which are bone-marrow (Robin) and leukaemia (Fox). I said goodbye to Maggie, the Sister there, who is getting a new job. Another nurse I know well is going to a children's hospice in the Southend area, as she lives there. She told me her fare, at the moment, is £300 a month. It also shows how dedicated and hard-working these nurses are to come such a long way. All the nurses at GOSH are super.

In Clarence I saw Natalie (C), 8, who was having her Achilles Tendon stretched, and Chantelle who has hip problems - she was born without hips.

In Nuffield CD I saw Erodotos. His Mum took our photo with Erodotos sitting on the arm of my chair, his arm round my shoulder. She gave me a box of Belgian chocolates from them all. In Alexandra I saw Mark (H) and Thomas; and Victoria (C) is back. Millie on the front desk told me there were two messages in my in-tray: they were from Pierre (H) and Karen (W).

Saturday October 28, Dolphin Square

Went to Chelsea to get two programmes, one for Emma and one for Ben. When I got back I found a devastating message which said:

This is Bridget Woollett down in Selling. I know you will be very sorry to hear that Alan Neame, who I know was a friend of yours, died yesterday evening. I don't know anything about any further arrangements, but I know you'll be sorry to hear about it. He had a massive stroke about a week ago and he's been unconscious ever since.

It was only about a month ago Alan telephoned me, and I didn't ring back as I intended writing to him, so he rang again and seemed anxious to know if I was OK. He's been a life-long friend since Oxford days, has been a good friend and helped me so much with my writing. I didn't see much of him in these later years but we kept in touch, and I will miss him a lot.

Later this evening I spoke to Iris, who lost Sean not long ago - about six weeks. She said everyone misses him, which of course they do. I also spoke to Annette. Little James is on 27 different drugs and medicines. Annette said she will make his next birthday, November 5, when he will be 7, a special one.

Sometimes something seems particularly sad, summing up the pathos of being a human being. On a TV programme this evening, which was about the Battle of Britain, a former Leading Seaman was talking of his experience on convoys. He said men from a sunken ship were swimming around in the middle of the ocean, and were waving to be picked up. But the Leading Seaman's ship charged through them to drop more depth charges and one man in the water, who knew he was going to die, kept calling out *Taxi Taxi*. The Leading Seaman remembers hearing the voice and the call *Taxi Taxi* fading. He said even strong men wept.

Had an email from Janice to say Scott was taken to GOSH on a doctor's emergency call (999 ambulance) to have his Baclofen pump turned off, as it was leaking and he wasn't getting the correct dosage. The drug was being leaked elsewhere in his body and making him swell up.

Took Ashley and Anya Kibblewhite to the Royal Mid-Surrey Golf Club for lunch. It was most enjoyable. They are such delightful company. Anya, who is Russian, is very attractive. We saw brother Alan and Wendy there and we all sat together for a little while and chatted. Then I went back to Ashley and Anya's mews house near Earl's Court which is full of expensive and lovely paintings and furniture; it is also large, on three floors. I looked at all the wedding photographs, which were so good. They gave me a beautiful one, large and mounted, with them and me in it.

Monday October 30, Dolphin Square

I took Elisabete O'Gorman, who works in the Dolphin Square Sports Centre, to GOSH today. She was caught in the worst storm we've had for a decade - two people killed, houses destroyed. She took two hours travelling (from Boreham Wood) for what is normally a twenty-minute journey. But she was OK getting back. She saw lots of children in different wards and got on well with them.

Fundraising told me that the Dolphin Square Sports Centre have sent in more GOSH collection boxes than anyone else. We owe it to Ronnie Page for this great effort.

Tuesday October 31, Dolphin Square

THE TIMES, TUESDAY OCTOBER 31, 2000

> NEAME - *Alan John only son of Alan Bruce and Annie Victoria Neame, late of Harefield Selling and dear friend and relation of many, died peacefully on 27th October after a short illness, aged 76. Cremation private. Requiem Mass at St Mary the Virgin Selling at 3pm 7th November. Family flowers only; donations if desired to The Stroke Association, Whitecross Street, London EC1Y 8JJ.*

Wednesday November 1, Dolphin Square

When I come to **Vision of Glory** I'll do it as if writing a letter. I have often rewritten a letter many times to get it right. Frank always said that this should be my approach to writing.

Thursday November 2, GOSH

I went into GOSH in the evening and saw quite a few of the children. Thomas was still in Alexandra Ward but going home tomorrow. Mark (H) had gone home. Little Yasmin was in isolation in Alexandra, sitting in a child's chair watching a Walt Disney and sucking her dummy, and with wires up her nose.She sleeps with her head in a large square glass case (like a fish bowl but square) as she is oxygen-dependent. She is so sweet and chatters away, although I can't make out what she's saying. Maureen, the Sister in Alexandra, told me what is wrong with Yasmin, it must be chest of some sort but I'll have to ask again. One of the nurses in Parrot said the children all love me and I certainly love them. I find a very strong bond of affection builds up with many of them.

Friday November 3, GOSH

A person called here this morning with remembrance poppies. I gave her 50p but I'm cynical about all that. Heroes in war but not wanted around too much in peace time.

Geraldine telephoned this morning. Danielle and Karl are in a sponsored swim for GOSH, so I've sent them £2.50 each for it.

Two very sad cases. Little George (P), is on a support line and, his father Tony told me, has only a few days to live. Tony and Suzanne want to take him home to die. Suzanne is expecting another baby soon. Because she had to have a test, to make sure the baby hasn't the same problem as George, she knows it will be a boy, and they are calling him Harry.

The other sad case is Joseph (C), aged 9, who has bone cancer. He is waiting for the result of a biopsy, but will have to go to the Middlesex Hospital for treatment. His parents are not all that hopeful of a full recovery. I said I would keep in touch, both with them and with George's parents.

Saturday November 4, Dolphin Square

This morning I had a letter from Geraldine sending me a copy of Barry's school reports which are very good. I also had a letter from Carol (F) to say Scott is coming into GOSH on 16th November; also one from Adam (K) giving me his news. And a letter from David Longbottom thanking me for two books on author's places (where they lived) which I gave him and Judy.

Sunday November 5, Dolphin Square

Marie (Everett), Rosie's daughter wrote:
*I have gone through **501 Days**, I quite liked it, but I wonder if it wouldn't have been a good idea if you condensed it by a quarter. You give some good advice for all, but it would be easier to get through if a little smaller........I did especially like your theme of 'Be what you are, and do what you think is right for yourself'.*
She is absolutely right. Excellent advice.

Ian's 65th birthday.

Monday November 6, Dolphin Square

Bobby called in this morning and put me onto Alliance Leicester banking facilities where I can earn interest. I'll keep Lloyds but use Alliance Leicester for my books.

Duke University Law Library, North Carolina, asked for a copy of **Violence** which I have sent.

Tuesday November 7, GOSH

Went into GOSH this afternoon to see Scott (R). He's had his operation to put his stomach pump right - it had been leaking.

I saw little Yasmin in Alexandra and gave her a lovely book of animals and birds in colour which I get from the London Zoological Society, as I'm a member.

I also saw Joseph (C). Cheryl, his Mum, was there, and Barbara, his Grandmother. His Grandfather, Seth, came in later. Joe is a very sick child; he has cancer in the spine and there are signs of secondaries in his chest. He was sedated by morphine, lying in bed. He goes to the Middlesex Hospital tomorrow for radio therapy: we don't do this at GOSH. I'll go and see him there. He is in awful pain and it seems the tumour is pressing on a nerve. In Dickens I saw Riza. She is always very bright.

I got some chocolate buttons for little Lewis (R); also chocolates for Victoria in Alexandra. Another friend of mine of quite long standing is Aleema in Transitional Care who smiled, and looked better. She has a major problem with breathing and has a tracheotomy.

In Lion I saw Scread (L). Her Mum, Risa, said she has a brain tumour. She has just come in so I'll see her again on Thursday. I also saw another old friend Saskia (B), who was in for the day. She is very well now but can't hear at all, and has to be told everything by sign language. She's about 6, I'm not sure of her age. She's a pretty little girl. I can't recall immediately what is wrong. It will be in my notebook. In Parrot I saw Christina (U), 13, who has aneurysm.

This evening I watched the Booker Prize entertainment. I remember Frank Jackson, a top critic, saying listen to four critics discussing the same work and you know what you are up against. It was just like that. One critic liked a book, another didn't like it; then they thought a first novel that had been short-listed should never have been there, and three of them (including Alain de Botton, whose excellent book on Proust I am reading) picked the winner who didn't win.

Wednesday November 8, Dolphin Square

6.00am news. The race between Al Gore and George Bush for U.S. President is still so tight that the result can't be at all certain.

9.00am news. Before this it said that Bush had got in as President. Now it says it's in doubt and Gore has retracted his admission of defeat.

10.00am news. They still don't know who the next President will be. I am quite sure it will be Mr George Bush.

Thursday November 9, GOSH

When I am dealing with very sick children, I find I lose all interest in who is going to be President of the United States (which hasn't yet been decided). I am always upset by children's illnesses, the serious ones we get at GOSH, but I don't let them take over emotionally, otherwise I couldn't do the job. But there are two patients whose illnesses I find very disturbing, because of the suffering it causes them. Emma (T) and Craig (M). Both have terrible skin complaints, and I mean terrible. Emma is home at the moment and she's reasonably cheerful, but Craig, 16, whom I saw this evening lying on his bed in Alice Ward, is covered, except for his shoulders, from head to foot in white bandages. He has a rare skin disease. All over his body are bright red sores. I only saw his shoulders, but since every other part of his body is bandaged I can only assume it's the same all over. He is a tall, slim, good-looking youngster who doesn't give away much in conversation and seems bitter, which is understandable. But whether it's me because he doesn't know me all that well, or whether he's the same with everyone, I don't know. He is leaving GOSH and going to St. Thomas's, because of his age. I would like to keep in touch with him. He said I could get his address from the nurses, so I'll have to see how things work out. But I do feel so deeply sorry for him, and for Emma.

Daniel (F) is in PICU, as his heart (transplant) is rejecting - I think that's what it is. I was able to go in and see him. He is very, very ill. I walked over to the Middlesex Hospital to see Joe who has started treatment. He was more lively, and didn't seem to be in pain though still hopping about because of the tumour pressing on a nerve. His Mother, Cheryl, wants to come back to GOSH and it is easy to see why. At GOSH Joe had his own room and much more fuss was made of him; but he must have his radium treatment there. The Sister in Lion Ward told me he could come back to Lion afterwards. He's a very affectionate boy.

I found out more about Yasmin in Alexandra Ward. She is 2+ years old and has chronic lung disease and oxygen-dependency. She is a lovely child. She kept saying *book, book* because of the book on animals and birds I had given her.

I saw also Janice and sat with her and Scott in Parrot Ward until 9.30pm.

Had a long talk to Inga about her work. She creates the most lovely mosaics.

Friday November 10, Dolphin Square

The diary for 2000 will be my last diary.

Saturday November 11, Dolphin Square

I've been feeling very down and sleepy, although better now (6.30pm). I'm sure the reason is my reaction to seeing Craig in Alice. It was a combination of the sort of bitter expression on his face (and who could blame him), and seeing this very good-looking youngster lying on his bed, bandaged all over, unable to do what normal teenagers do: play football, go to dances etc. I don't know why he has so disturbed me; if it happened often I couldn't do the job. It must be symbolic of all the sadness involved with very ill children.

Today people have stood for two minutes silence for the war dead. I know we had to go to war, but I'm a bit cynical about some of it, this nonsense about laying down your life. You don't, on the whole, lay down your life deliberately; it's taken from you. I've said all this before.

Bridget Woollett telephoned this evening. She had been to Alan Neame's funeral. Very sad. I can't believe he's not there. We'd been close friends for so many years. I'll miss him as I do Freddie Ludlow.

Sunday November 12, Dolphin Square

I was told yesterday that Alan, at the beginning of the war, worked in the Secret Service, and that he was an Army Captain at 21. A sort of delayed shock has set in and I find it difficult not to think of him still at Selling.

Today I wrote to Anna (G), who was Sister in Alice Ward, about my problem over Craig. She is now on maternity leave. I'll take the letter into GOSH on Tuesday and get them to forward it. This is what I wrote:

Dear Anna

Excuse me typing this, but my handwriting is not all that good. I wanted to ask your advice.

During the 5+ years I have been working at the hospital (the last three ward-visiting) I have dealt, obviously, with many sick children and, sadly, children who have died. In some cases the parents asked me to be with the children at the end. I wouldn't be human if seeing sick children didn't make me feel sad, but I have coped, looking upon it that if I can bring some comfort to parents and children it is worth it.

However, on Thursday evening last week, I went in to see Craig (M), in Alice. You may have dealt with him when you were Sister there. He is 16 and is leaving GOSH because of his age, to go to St Thomas's Hospital.

I can't fully explain, but I felt deeply disturbed when I saw him, bandaged from his shoulders to his feet with this terrible skin complaint. I could see some of it. He was lying there looking really fed up (I would almost say bitter) and I felt an overwhelming pity, thinking what a normal fine-looking teenager would be doing - such as playing football, going to parties etc.

He wasn't very communicative and didn't want to give me his home address, only said he lived in Brighton and I could ask the nurses for it. I would have liked to have kept in touch with him, as I do with many children who write to me here. It's something that's built up with the job.

I only felt as disturbed as this on one other occasion, when I was working as a volunteer in a terminal hospice (Dr Cecily Saunders) where there was a young man of 24 paralysed from the neck down - he couldn't use any part of his body and was trapped in it, but was mentally alert. He was very bitter and was hostile, even to his young wife. I got this feeling with Craig, that he was trapped, which may have been because he was so heavily bandaged and didn't seem to be able to move.

What I do with many children is get them sweets (with permission of course) and some I send a birthday card with a £5 note. It means a lot to them, and it's not me being generous, because I doubt if I spend more than £300 a year on the children, and I don't lead any sort of social life as I'm too busy with my work here and at GOSH. You can spend five times that amount on one trip abroad.

I would like to write to Craig and send him £5 for his birthday - he is 16 on 20 October - but I don't really know what to do. On only two occasions I have been asked by parents not to visit their child and have fully understood, but I didn't get any sort of rejection from Craig, although I haven't met his parents.

This is the situation, and I would be grateful for your advice.

I hope you don't mind my writing about this, but I would like to try and find out why I have felt as I did, and what I should do about it.

Monday November 13, Dolphin Square

Saw Mr Georgeou about my teeth. He is an excellent Dentist. Bobby goes to him, too. I'm on National Health, but it's not cheap. £61 today. I saw Francine in reception and we spoke about her children.

Iris and Michael sent me a copy of Sean's funeral service, beautifully done with a coloured photo of Sean on the front page. Very sad. He was adored by all. Iris and Michael, who had adopted him, were so loving and caring as were all the family.

This morning I went to Lloyds in Pall Mall. It reminded me of the good old days when Derek Collins was the Pall Mall Manager and I used to go and have lunch with him in the Bank's dining room. Stephanie Black, the Business Banking Manager, who has set up the business company for me, told me that they can take a client out to lunch but first have to fill in a form answering 50 questions. There was also a very nice young man there, Neil Price, a graduate trainee.

Had my usual Monday sitting with Bill. His portrait of me is very good.

Isobel telephoned this evening. I am going to see her and John for lunch on 27 December, which will be very nice.

Tuesday November 14, GOSH

I went to GOSH and took flowers for Stephen (C). I put them in the chapel. Noel and Jill got a nice vase. The flowers were white and pink (reddish pink) carnations. Then I went to Alice but Craig had gone home. In Alexandra I saw little Yasmin, and Chelsea.

Daniel (F) has been moved from PICU to CICU. He is very, very ill. I spoke to his Dad, Lew, who is pessimistic about his chances of recovery. I didn't speak about him to Kathy, his Mum. His heart has packed up and he is on a pump; he also has a clot of blood and his kidneys have failed. It will be a miracle if he survives. I'll see him - if he is still there - on Friday.

In PICU I saw Karima (G) who had been knocked down by a bus. Her Mum, Mafedha, said Karima had run in front of it, and until today has been in a coma. When I saw her she had just opened her eyes. Her elder brother, Khalid, was with her. Mafedha told me her husband died seven years ago. He must have been quite young. What is worrying for everyone at the moment is that they don't know the extent of Karima's injuries, especially to her head.

Rita rang me this morning. Her son, Richard, who is in America, is giving two of my books, **Violence** and **The Trial** to Kentucky University library, where he was a student.

Wednesday November 15, Dolphin Square

Had a long email from Byron.

Bought Yasmin a card with a kitten on it and posted it to her at GOSH.

Bill came here and I typed two letters for him.

Thursday November 16, Dolphin Square

Andy and Jane, Ali and Anita came to the Golf Club this evening for dinner. It was very pleasant. Saw Ted and Glen there, both looking well.

Friday November 17, GOSH

Went to CICU to see Daniel. He is still very, very ill, but there is a slight improvement as I think his kidneys are working a little. Kathy is with him. He dozes off, then opens his eyes and dozes off again. He had just had his oxygen tube removed but is still on the heart pump. It was his birthday on 11th, he was 13 so I got him a birthday card.

In Parrot I saw Karima (G) who is now conscious. She left PICU, but is very confused. She won't eat. Khalid, her brother, was trying to get her to eat and I could see I was more in the way than helping so I left, and went to the other side of the ward to see Matthew (D),10, who had been operated on that morning for a brain tumour. He was lying asleep with the top of his head in a bandage. His parents, Paul and Sandra, look young to have a boy of 10. They are a charming couple but naturally very worried about Matthew. Next to Matthew I saw Darren (W),14. He'd had an operation on his brain to stop him having fits. His Mum told me the operation had been successful and he wasn't now getting fits. I spoke to him a little, a delightful boy. The operation hadn't affected his intelligence: he was OK in this respect.

In Alexandra I saw Chelsea and gave her 50p to buy whatever she wants. Her Mum was with her. Just along the corridor I saw Yasmin. She was wandering about attached to a long plastic blue line that was fixed to a machine. I'm not sure what it was for. She showed me the card with the picture of the kitten I had sent her. She's lovely. I saw Ismail in Fox and gave his Mum the white chocolate buttons he asked for.

In the canteen Emma (L) came up to thank me for my birthday card. Her boy friend David was with her. He is 20, very nice. He works in the hospital, too. Emma is looking for another job to get more money and experience.

Lydia (N) was leaving in a wheelchair with her father, a nurse pushing her, to go to UCH. She's an old friend of mine. She looked ill, and said she was feeling bad. She had been to Robin, which is the leukaemia ward (bone marrow transplant). I have her home address so will write to her this weekend.

In Victoria I saw George (P), 10. He's had a kidney problem which was why he was in Victoria, but his major problem is Lymphoma, and he is actually a Lion Ward patient. Lion is a cancer ward. In Lion I saw Michael (S) who is staff and works in the ward. He is very nice and got me the home address of Darren (P), as I wanted to write and thank Darren's Mum for the note she left. While I was talking to Michael, Alex came up. He is young and delightful and is also staff.

Saturday November 18, Dolphin Square

I've been working most of today on the proof of Volume Four of the diaries. Redwood and Peter Holloway who looks after me, are excellent.

I forgot to mention yesterday that I had quite a long chat to Rita as she was on duty in the Italian. She is very kindly taking copies of **Violence** and **The Trial** to America when she goes in December (she and Roy have an apartment in Florida) to give to her son Richard, who is going to give them to Kentucky University library. Rita is a very kind person.

Sunday November 19, Dolphin Square

Just telephoned CICU and spoke to Kathy. Daniel is still holding his own and his kidneys have improved a little although there is still some fluid on his lungs. He's back on the oxygen tube, and also continuing with his heart pump.

Today I finished the corrections - the final ones - for Volume Four of the diaries.

This afternoon I saw *The Battle of Midway* on TV. It didn't get a good write-up - poor construction etc. - but it brought back haunting memories of the *Malaya*, and how we were going into battle with the German battlecruiser, and the terror I felt. I felt so much for the American pilots in this respect. I'm not sure about the Japanese: they are so cold-blooded. I don't know if they feel anything.

Ben telephoned this morning. He had tried to get me last weekend. We had quite a long chat and I was very pleased to hear from him and to learn he was very well - good news.

Monday November 20, Dolphin Square

Had a sitting with Bill.

Tuesday November 21, GOSH

Came back from GOSH this afternoon and at about 6.20pm Annette telephoned to say that she had been told by the local hospital, where James had been, that the little boy was so ill nothing more could be done and that all treatment should be withdrawn. Annette refused to sign her consent to this, and took him home. She said in the years to come she would feel much better about it- if there is any feeling of betterness in such an agonising situation - if she did all she could, as long as he's not in pain, to keep him with her and the family. So I said she should do this, after all she is his mother. Doctors are very caring and I am sure their decision was made for the best motives, but I can see it as almost impossible for a mother to sign such a consent.

At GOSH today I saw Lydia (C), 4, who has leukaemia. Marian Charlesworth had written to tell me about her, as Lydia is the God-daughter of one of Marian's church friends. I met Kate, Lydia's Mum, and Lydia's Grandmother.

I saw little Yasmin in Alexandra, who was lying with her head in her glass oxygen case, also Chelsea.

I gave Ismail, in Fox, some more white chocolate buttons. In CICU I saw Daniel. He was able to talk but with effort. There is a meeting on him this afternoon, with the possibility of him having another heart transplant.

I bumped into Jacob's (H) Mum, Nina. They are going home, which is great news. Jacob had, I think, leukaemia; at any rate he was in that ward (Fox). Baby Noah, a few weeks old, in CICU, is still holding his own. He's tiny.

I saw Emma and David by the front desk. I like Emma very much, and David. There is a lovely Chinese girl called La working behind the front desk. Everyone likes her.

Wednesday November 22, Dolphin Square

Bridget Woollett sent this cutting from the local Kent paper, with a copy of the funeral service:

FUNERAL OF WRITER AND TRANSLATOR.

AN AUTHOR and linguist who translated religious works and served as an intelligence officer during the Second World War has died at the age of 76.

Alan Neame, a bachelor of Vicarage Lane, Selling, was cremated at Charing following a full requiem mass at St Mary the Virgin, Selling on Thursday.

Although he wrote two novels in the 1960s - The Adventures of Maud Noakes and Maud Noakes, Guerrilla - Mr Neame was known for his religious works.

A biography on Elizabeth Barton, the Holy Maid of Kent was followed by a translation of the psalms in the Jerusalem Bible from Latin into English.

Mr Neame also translated Italian scientific papers on the Turin Shroud into English.

He was president of the East Kent Historical Society and a keen genealogist.

Educated at Cheltenham College and Wadham College, Oxford, Mr Neame joined the Intelligence Corps in 1943 and studied Japanese at Bletchley Park.

Posted to the Far East, he was mentioned in dispatches for work carried out behind Japanese lines and became a captain at the age of 21.

After the war he taught at Cheltenham College before going to the Middle East where he worked as a teacher in Cairo and Baghdad.

Thursday November 23, Dolphin Square

Bridget Woollett wrote about Alan:
It is very sad for all of us in the village. He was always supportive at occasions such as charity coffee morning, the summer fete etc. and had also compiled a very interesting and readable history of Selling Church. Although he was extremely clever and talented he never made one feel conscious of this, but always had time to make one laugh! I know you will miss him very much too.
(Written 19 November)

Friday November 24, Dolphin Square

I had to be at Moorfields for an 8.30am appointment. Dr Keegan, whom I had had before, examined me and said that, although my eyes will deteriorate, unless something drastic happens it will be very gradual, because what I have at the back of my eye is benign. He said that by the time I am 112 (to use his own words) my sight will have been very much affected. I have been going every four months, but now I haven't to go back for another nine months for a check-up, in August next year.

I like Dr Keegan very much, as I do all the doctors at Moorfields, but have been fortunate to have the same doctors. I've had a charming Spanish lady doctor several times. Moorfields is an excellent eye hospital, so efficient and caring.

The Parker 51 fountain pen Bobby sent me from Hong Kong, when he was a Royal Marine officer there during the war has, after almost sixty years of constant use (used for all my writing - novels etc.), come to an end. I was hoping to finish this diary, still using it, but I've tried and tried, and it will go reasonably well for a short time, then start scratching, and it's then difficult to write. So I'll clean it and put it away. It's been a marvellous pen for all this time.

After Moorfields I went into GOSH. I saw Dan. He is still so ill. He is just 13 and lies asleep, in his prettily patterned hospital shirt, the tube going into his mouth, his breathing not very jerky, but not even, his arms by his side, his hands closed. It is so sad seeing him like this - it is devastating for Kathy - her only child. He has a lock of fair hair falling boyishly over his forehead. It seems his kidneys have picked up a little but there is so much wrong, his heart is so damaged and, although he's been put on the emergency list for another heart, even when one is found he may be too ill for the transplant.

I also visited baby Noah - so tiny -who is making good progress. Lydia (G), 4, has moved down to Fox which is the leukaemia ward. She has started treatment and had sick bouts yesterday, but this is what the treatment does. There are ups and downs right the way through.

Little Yasmin was in bed with her head in her glass case, and as she was about to go to sleep I didn't stop long.

I bumped into David, a young volunteer, and I was pleased when he told me that he does exactly what I do, building up relationships with parents and children, and writing to them at Christmas. He covers the three cardiac wards. It has often been on my conscience that I don't cover these wards enough, but now I know I don't need to.

Emily (S) came in, and I persuaded her to let me give her a birthday present; she never will let me buy her anything when she comes to GOSH for a check-up. I'm very fond of her. She has to use crutches all the time.

Inga was in the Italian, so I saw her twice and we had, as always, interesting conversations. We were both surprised that Robert

Creighton, the Chief Executive, had left in four days. The Chairman, Naomi Sargent, too, had gone suddenly and Lois also, who was a Trustee. Dave King, our Fire Officer, is also going. I was sorry to hear this. Dave is one of the nicest people you could meet and has been here a long time.

At 5.00pm Salina came and collected me. First I took her up to see Kathy (F) whom Salina knew well, and also Dan. But the doctors were operating in CICU so we couldn't go in. I left Salina with Kathy in the waiting room.

A little later I went out to where Roy was waiting in the car. Emma and David came out and we talked for a little while, then I went with Salina and Roy to their flat in Islington and spent the evening there. They gave me the most delicious dinner and we had a long gossip about GOSH; it was most enjoyable.

They insisted on bringing me back here, so they came up for a few minutes and I gave them Volumes Two and Three of my diaries, and I gave Roy the Cow & Gate booklet as he was very interested. I'm very fond of Salina and Roy is very nice. A super evening.

Saturday November 25, Dolphin Square

For most of today I've been working on my disc for Volume Five of the diaries. I have finished it and will post it off to Peter by first post Monday.

Sunday November 26, Dolphin Square

Had a long chat to Bobby on the telephone.

I've started on Volume Six of the diaries, putting in Rhoda's corrections. I rang her up this morning to see how she was, and she is feeling better.

Anna hasn't replied to my letter of 12 November (on Craig) but Bobby said there's probably a very simple reason; she's too busy with two small children. He said there's a saying in the church: don't look for a supernatural reason before seeking an ordinary one.

Monday November 27, Dolphin Square

Had a long sitting with Bill for my portrait.

Tuesday November 28, Dolphin Square

Fiona telephoned this evening. Her baby is now 14 days old and is called Charlie Weinel Davies.

Wednesday November 29, Dolphin Square

Anna telephoned this morning and gave me the full picture on Craig, and it did help me a lot. She said he has an appalling skin disease and all the staff dealing with him find it disturbing and depressing because it affects him so badly. Anna has laid it on that I can write to Craig through Yvette or Jackie, Alice nurses. I'll send him £10 for his birthday, and if he doesn't reply I'll let it go. But he's coming back to GOSH even though he's over age, and the nurses will let me know when he's in. I do appreciate Anna telephoning; it's been a great help.

I had an email from Inga and it summed up beautifully what Bill had said to me in the painting room. I showed the email to Bill and he felt, as I did, that it was so beautifully composed. This is what Inga wrote:

Dear William - I think your friend is right. Everyone has their own way of coping with difficulties. The important thing is that you are there when they need you most and that is in the hospital. What happens afterwards, when they return to the lives which were interrupted by illness or death, is something else and maybe they don't want to keep in touch with that part of their lives - it is too painful.

You are not part of the painful time although you are the relief, the person who helps them get through at the time. I do not pretend to understand this process but, I can see that it is complex. One thing I am sure of and that is the fact that your presence, interest and care for the children is of the utmost importance.

People do not on the whole keep in touch with doctors or nurses, in spite of the vital care they give, for any longer than they have to. It does not mean they do not appreciate what they have done. It is just that people do not want to be reminded of illness or death when they are back home. It is a time of trauma, being dislocated from home and away from loved ones often for long periods of time. I am sure they think back with gratitude that there was someone who cared enough to talk to them and their children at a most difficult time in their lives.

You meet such a lot of children and parents that it is impossible for you to keep up contact with them all for ever - maybe you have to accept that you are doing your best work in the Hospital itself and that once they have left they fall back on their own support network and your job is done until they come back again, if they do.

The thing is that human beings are erratic and their reactions incomprehensible, illogical and thoroughly annoying!!!!

I bumped into Bill this afternoon and we were talking about Malcolm Bradbury who has just died at 65. Bill said he was a good story-teller. Bill said he also did a lot of his classes in the local pub and authors would bring in their plots. I told Bill I'd done this at the City Lit and found it a waste of time. I recalled to Bill the classes I went to which Ian Cochrane took. Ian, who had published a couple of funny novels, was very nice. But after a while he didn't turn up, so I took over the rest of the classes for that term and got paid for it.

A very nice young man who lives here, Gordon Rae, has just come up. I bumped into him in the lift. He has shown me how to take copy of a floppy disc. He is just under me on the fourth floor.

This morning, in the shower room, I was talking to Michael Shaw, and was telling him about my interview with Lord Butler when I was writing about Forsyth. Michael knew Butler well and told me that he had it in his grasp to become Prime Minister, but he couldn't stop talking, and gave confidential information to the press and so on. I found this very interesting.

Thursday November 30, GOSH

So much has happened today, I'll take it in order of everything happening rather than importance because, obviously, most important of all are the GOSH children.

I had a letter from Marjorie Baker. She and Jodie had been to Northampton to see where Cyril had lived and had been brought up, and I found the description moving:

Jodie and I went out with an A-Z street map to find the address where Cyril had been fostered from July 1936 till September 1941 by a Mr and Mrs Robbins. It is the one place he could remember well and had fond memories of going on holidays with the Robbins. Unfortunately Mrs Robbins became ill and was taken into hospital and so they had to be moved.

We found the house, which looked very much as I imagine it looked sixty years ago and just across the road was the park that Cyril talked about. It was all very moving. We also found St James School still standing just around the corner, but being the school holidays the gates were locked so we had to be content with the view from the road. Jodie was so pleased we had been able to find so much from her Grandfather's past still there. As you say Barnardo's has made such a difference to lots of lives. Cyril

*always said he was happy with Barnardo's and told Mr Smith
who brought his file up from London, when he was going through
it with him.*

Then I had an email from the mother of a GOSH teenager who
had been very ill and fortunately is much better. He had also
written to me, but the mother's email was full of problems. She
had lost her teenage niece, whom I saw in GOSH, and who later
died from cancer. I have said often there is nothing worse than
losing a child, it is devastating and the loss is always there.

I got to GOSH in the morning, had a very nice lunch in the staff
canteen and went over to the Italian to see Rita who was on the
reception desk. I had given her a copy of **Violence** (as she had
given a copy to her son to give to Kentucky University) and to my
surprise she said once she started reading it she couldn't put it
down; then her family read it and they felt the same. She said
she found the first half particularly interesting because it was
about me, my life in the Navy, in the war and so on. I knew she
meant what she said because she asked questions on incidents in
the book, the rebellious butler and other characters. I was
surprised because it is not an easy book to read; in fact I think it
is very difficult.

I went to see Dan and found that he had had a second heart
transplant. He was on the emergency list and it was done
quickly, because without it he wouldn't have lived. I was able to
see him through the window of the transplant room in DJW.

Lew, his father, came out (Kathy had gone home for a short
break) and he told me they had left the decision to Dan, whether
or not he would go through with the second transplant. He was
aware that if he didn't he wouldn't have lived for more than a few
days; but he might have wanted to die rather than go through all
the trauma of another transplant. But Dan decided to have it so
we are all hoping so much that he will get permanently better.
I'll see him when I go in next week.

Then I saw Jimmy (W), 14, whom I have seen before, when he
came in to have a tumour removed from the upper part of his leg.
Unfortunately another tumour has come back in the same place
and naturally his parents, and everyone, are very worried. It is a
rare tumour, but doesn't seem to be malignant. Jimmy has had a
scan, but it's too soon for results so I'll know more about it the
next time I see him.

Alison, who is in the Italian Hospital and works in fundraising,
gave me a lovely toy tiger which I took to Alexandra and gave to

Yasmin. She was very pleased. The nurses are trying to get her out of sucking her dummy all the time, so she tried to get me to get it for her; I asked the nurse but was told they want to try and get her out of the habit as she is 2+. I saw other children so didn't leave until 8.30pm.

In the evening I watched a fascinating programme on the universe. Astronomers have discovered that black holes, the most destructive force in space, are at the centre of each galaxy of which ours is in the Milky Way. Scientists have calculated that in three billion years time the earth will collide with (I think) the Milky Way which, although it looks like stars strung out, is a huge round disc, that there will be the most almighty explosion, everything destroyed, with the earth no more than a piece of burnt toast. I believe it, because if scientists can calculate how to put man on the moon, placing the rocket there on time to a second, they can get it right about the earth. So what does it all add up to, and where is God?

Friday December 1, Dolphin Square

I finished the floppy disc for Volume Six of my diaries. Gordon Rae showed me how to make copies of the disc.

Geraldine telephoned and we made arrangements for me to go out tomorrow. I am going to see Danielle and Karl in their swimming gala and am looking forward to it.

Saturday December 2, Dolphin Square

This morning on the news I heard that British prisoners-of-war, taken by the Japanese are to get £10,000 each as compensation for their sufferings; but Gurka soldiers who fought for Britain, and were also Japanese prisoners-of-war are to get nothing. This proves the hypocrisy of all this war hero business. Faced with the choice how many would volunteer to lay down their life? Not very many. You lose your life and that's a matter of chance. In action, in the Mediterranean, I didn't see anyone who was all that keen on getting killed, in fact the opposite. We were all petrified. I've already mentioned the government trying to get out of continuing with war widows' pensions and, although we couldn't let Hitler take over, that when the need for heroism has passed so has general concern for the heroes.

In 1985, when I had just had my 66th birthday (I saw this in a diary), Lionel asked me which age I enjoyed the most and I said now, at the age I was then. Recently Rita asked me the same question and I gave the same answer, the age I am now, 81, this has been one of the happiest years of my life.

10.00pm. Just got back from an evening with the Stapletons. I went to see Danielle and Karl competing in their annual swimming gala. It was a lovely evening. Danielle won two gold medals and one silver, Karl four gold medals and one silver. Kieran was home and Kevin came in from playing tennis. Barry had been to watch Arsenal who beat Southampton 1-0. He came to the pool, but went out again to a friend's birthday party. Geraldine has asked me out tomorrow for Christmas lunch.

Sunday December 3, Dolphin Square

I went to see the Stapletons again today. Geraldine had an early Christmas lunch as they are going to their house in Ireland. Kieran was there, and Danielle and Karl. Barry was working in Waitrose. Kevin came in later as he had been playing tennis. Afterwards Karl came with Geraldine to take me to the station. The meal was delicious.

Rita rang this evening. I'm seeing her at GOSH on 14th, then we'll fix up to meet when she comes back from her apartment in Florida, where she and Roy are going for Christmas.

Monday December 4, Dolphin Square

Stuart Sampson, who is very high up in the Crown Prosecution Service, also lectures on the First World War. He is very knowledgeable and interesting. I meet him in the pool most mornings and enjoy talking to him.

Tuesday December 5, Dolphin Square

Went into Marks (Pantheon) this morning and saw Lily, Charmaine, Liz, Rosie, Cathy, Kathy, Yvette, Laura, Pam, Audrey, Yasmin, Juanita, Tian, Zoran, Sam, James.

Had another bulletin from John Hipkin on the awfulness of teenage soldiers being executed for 'cowardess' in the First World War. No excuse for these brutal acts, and certainly, long ago, there should have been a general pardon.

Very interesting. On TV this evening it showed pictures from archives, of Japanese survivors (you don't often get it this way round). One Japanese survivor said that when they were being killed by the Americans, none mentioned the Emperor; they did call their mother's names, but as the Emperor was responsible for a million Japanese soldiers dying, why did he not accept some responsibility? I could tell the Japanese survivor why, because he was the Emperor and, like the Kaiser in the First World War, should have been hanged. But they never do accept, or are not allowed to accept, responsibility for the evil they do.

Wednesday December 6, Dolphin Square

Saw another documentary on TV today about children who survived the German concentration camps, and were rootless and lost. Terrible.

The Guardian has pages on Britain becoming a republic and why the institution of monarchy is no longer working, and that British people prefer to be citizens rather than subjects.

Had an interesting letter from Anne Huibregtse who lives in America. She wrote about a woman in a car accident whose three-year-old daughter was killed, then the mother miscarried and lost the child she was expecting. Anne said she didn't know how the woman coped. I met Anne at the Doubledays; she knew Edwin well. She is a very clever sculptor.

Thursday December 7, Dolphin Square

Went to Bexhill and had a delicious lunch with Peter and Daphne Studd. I always enjoy my visits to them. Peter is 85 on 2 March, and Daphne 80 in February. They were both looking very well. Memories of Maud (Bill Lundon's mother) always come back, not that I need any prompting to remember her or Bill.

Spoke to Geraldine this evening. She's caught a cold and sore throat so wasn't feeling too good. I also spoke to Danielle, who was very pleased as she's got a day off from school.

Had a very nice Christmas present from Byron: a beautiful and attractive scarf.

Also a Christmas card from Barbara Warner telling me about the party of 120 which they had for Ned's 90th birthday.

Friday December 8, GOSH

Got to GOSH at 11.00am and took another collection box from Ronnie Page. Hayley, in Fundraising, sent him a lovely picture of GOSH children, which is framed and on the sports centre reception desk by the box.

Then I had a chat to Inga, who was on duty in the Italian. It is always interesting and enjoyable talking to her. In my in-tray were letters and cards from Kathy and Jimmy. Jimmy wrote:

Dear William

I am writing to tell you how I feel about my illness and when I am in hospital. My illness is called Polyarteritis Nodosa which affects the medium size blood vessels which can cause them to pop. Unfortunately one popped in my leg and caused me to have an operation to clear the lump. When they sent the lump to be analysed they found a rare tumour called Angiomatied Fibrous Histlolytoma which was not cancerous thankfully. My immune system has been suppressed and so I cannot really get in contact with any colds, diseases and bugs. I am on steroids to keep the illness calm, and tablets.

I don't really mind being in hospital because the nurses look after you well and have a laugh with you and the doctors do normally get you well quite quickly. Since I have been ill I haven't felt that bad about it, of course I would rather be well and playing football like I used to and playing other sports which I miss too. I haven't been to school for about 18 months which is quite a long while but I have been having a home tutor and they are both nice to me. I hope I get well soon so I can get back to my usual things and be good at football again, from Jimmy Warner.

As usual I saw a lot of children. Dan has improved, but when I say this it is relative: his new heart saved his life, which was hanging by a thread because his first heart (the transplanted one) was so damaged. He is still very ill and has only been able to get out for a very short time in a wheelchair. But he is out of the transplant room, and in an ordinary one. He is a brave boy who, as I've said before, has been through so much. Of course the stress is not only his, but falls heavily on his parents. When I was in his room two doctors, a man and a lady, were examining his chest by running a tube with a rubber end (it looked like this) over him, so that a black and white image of his heart beating appeared on a screen. The Senior Doctor, the man, said his heart was perfectly all right but there was fluid in his diaphragm. I do hope he pulls through and this heart doesn't reject. I don't think he can take much more going wrong.

Some of the children I saw last time have gone home but I meet new ones. Christopher (M) in RBC has a heart and lung condition. He is 15 and has been coming into GOSH since he was a baby. His legs are very swollen due to fluid, which they are trying to disperse by medication. He then has to have an operation which is overdue - not the hospital's fault.

My little friend Yasmin was in Alexandra. She was walking about with lines attached to her and was very bright and chatted away to me. I gave her a book with cats and dogs in it (Paws from Battersea Dogs Home). She loves animal books.

Jonathan, 13, in Giraffe has a very low immune system. He has so much wrong with him including internal bleeding. Little Harry (B), 4 months, in Lion Ward has Neuroblastoma. I saw Maggie, who was one of the Sisters in Robin and Fox but she has left GOSH and is doing supply work as a nurse. It was very nice seeing her again but she was very busy and couldn't stop. I also saw Lindy, the Sister in Parrot Ward. I like her, and all the Sisters and Nurses I know.

Emma was working in Elephant Day Care. She told me she has a new job and is leaving at the end of the month.

I was supposed to be meeting Nicky in GOSH, but had an email from Sam (his Mum) to say she didn't feel well enough to bring him as she's just has a Caesarian for her new baby; they will be coming again in January.

When I got back I had a message on my answering machine from Peter Holloway giving me news of my diaries, which are coming along well.

Saturday December 9, Dolphin Square

I had breakfast here with brother Ian and Margaret, as they are staying in a guest room. It was very nice seeing them. Margaret's knee is much better.

This afternoon I watched again *The Sinking of the Bismark*. Stiff upper lip propaganda making out fighting and killing is glorious. Nothing like reality.

Betty telephoned this evening and we had a long chat. Very nice. I'm going to see Ali and Anita on 29th. Andy and Jane are abroad on two weeks holiday.

Sunday December 10, Dolphin Square

I've spent all day writing (mostly) to GOSH children. I've got everything cleared up.

Monday December 11, Dolphin Square

My diary cover for Volume Four came from Peter Holloway this morning. It's very good, with a photo of *HMS Malaya* on the back.

Tuesday December 12, GOSH

Went into GOSH today to see David (H) who came in for a check-up. He looked very bright and well. He is a delightful boy. He has written a ten-page autobiography which he is going to send me, and I'll put it, or part of it, in this diary. He had cancer of the bladder; the whole bladder was removed and a new bladder constructed. Thank goodness all is working well.

Noel, our Chaplain sent me the very sad news via Patti that Scott (R) died today. I think it was this morning. It was a shock as I hadn't expected it. I wrote to Janice.

Saw Samira (A) who had come in to see William Harkness for a check-up. She's had so many problems, poor little girl, but she seemed OK. I think she's had thirteen operations.

Saw little Yasmin in Alexandra. She's in isolation again as she has an infection, so you have to put on an apron and gloves before going into her room.

Dan is much better. He is sitting up and talking but is still very ill. I do hope he fully recovers and doesn't have another rejection. The food in the canteen is very good.

Saw Christopher in RBC. He hadn't had a very good night and wasn't all that good. Later I saw his mother taking him along the corridor in a wheelchair. He looked a little better.

I bumped into William Harkness in the corridor. He's a bit fed up because his mother (June) won't go to Spain and stay with them for Christmas. I told William I would speak to his mother, but I don't know if it will do any good.

In Marks (Pantheon) Yasmin (who works in foods) showed me photos of her new-born baby - very sweet.

Wednesday December 13, GOSH

This is taken from David's autobiography called:

MY SECOND CHANCE

Shortly after my third birthday I was diagnosed with a rare childhood cancer called Rhabdomyosarcoma. I had a lot of treatment over a year in Great Ormond Street Hospital including Chemotherapy and Radiotherapy. The treatment failed and I had to undergo a huge operation to remove my bladder. After the operation I became much stronger and increased my body weight by over a third in six months.

I told my Mum that I wanted to climb the highest mountain in England before my sixth birthday. My Mum thought I would forget about my wish soon but the idea had been born and I continued to think about Scafell Pike and what it would be like to be standing on the summit and being the highest person in England.

During the Easter holidays in 1995 we went on a self-catering holiday to a cottage in Ambleside. In the last few days before the holidays we packed up and watched the long-range weather forecast. This suggested that my dream could be fulfilled and that the first two days would have the best weather. The date for my ascent was set for Sunday 9th April 1995. The date was the second anniversary of me being in remission from the cancer. In all a party of nine set off on the walk at ten o'clock. I think that every one else was more serious than me and I can remember feeling excited and just knowing that I would be able to make it.

The first mile or so out of the valley was fairly easy going but soon afterwards it became trickier and more like a scramble. We stopped for a picnic about five metres below the snow line and I had an orange mug full of steaming mushroom soup and a peanut butter sandwich. It tasted so good and I can remember feeling the warmth trickle down my insides. After climbing a few more metres I found a sheet of snow and soon I started to 'ski' down on my boots. A great friend of the family 'Big John' lent me his ski pole so I could look the part. Soon the weather closed in and it became very misty but nevertheless we reached the summit in three and a half hours. At the top I felt disappointed at first and wasn't sure why. Then it dawned on me that my ambition was not just to be at the summit, but also to be the highest person in England. I asked Big John, the tallest member of the group, to lift me onto his shoulders and then I was completely happy.

A few days later the summit team got together for a celebration meal and my Uncle Peter presented me with a wonderful souvenir of a picture of Scafell Pike signed by Chris Bonnington. It is one of my prized possessions and hangs proudly on my bedroom wall. The day had also made history as we had three generations at the top including my Grandad who was sixty-seven. I didn't know at the time but my younger brother was also there with me as Mum was nine weeks pregnant.

People sponsored me for the 'expedition' and eventually I raised £12,500 which I gave to charities that help children with cancer. I was thrilled to be able to help and shall never forget the feeling at the top, which was a mixture of excitement and joy. The cairn at the top of Scafell Pike is one of the most remote and beautiful places and is definitely one of my favourites.

One person, outside the family, who has influenced me most is Olwyn Summers whom I met in 1999. At the time I was contemplating huge reconstructive surgery at Great Ormond Street Hospital. She was my form teacher and the Deputy Head Teacher at my Junior School. Olwyn influenced me by being the first person outside the family who tried to understand how much the operation meant to me and also how hard the decision was. For the first time in my life the decision was entirely mine and yet I knew all that lay ahead, the long period in hospital and the uncertainty of how I would feel afterwards. She helped me to overcome these fears and to concentrate on the 'pros' rather than the 'cons' of the operation. I went for the operation and she was very pleased for me and promised that she would visit me in hospital afterwards.

Many weeks later, the day came for the final tube to be taken out and as Dad was away on business I asked specifically if Olwyn could be there with my Mum to see me for the first time in eight years when I would have no tubes or bags on me externally. She witnessed the 'taking out of the tube' in the medical room at Gerrards Cross School. I really appreciate and admire her for that.

Ten weeks after I came out of hospital, year six (from school) went on an outward-bound course at the River Dart. In the weeks beforehand we did circuit training in the hall at school every morning before school to get fit. At the beginning I could hardly do anything and was put in the least fit group, which was Group 8 out of 8. One afternoon in the Games lesson we were doing 'Bleep Tests' and running between markers as quickly as we could. I did my best while she and Mum carried my bags and tubes. As always she was anxious I was trying too hard but was very supportive. I grew stronger and I was moved up through the groups. Olwyn was often there to encourage and praise me along with my schoolmates.

Having a desire, a hope or a dream is very important in life and if you try hard enough then you will nearly always succeed and fulfil your ambition. In the short term I hope to create new aspirations that I will strive to complete over time.

I was given a 'Second Chance' when I was three by Mr Duffy, a Consultant at Great Ormond Street, when he took out the tumour or 'naughty lump' (as it was called then) which could have killed me. I hope to make the best of his handiwork and not waste this brilliant chance.

My biggest desire is that when I am nearing the end of my life I will be able to look back and say that I have taken the most out of it and have very few regrets and have not wasted opportunities that I may have had. If I am able to say that, I will be the happiest person alive.

Thursday December 14, GOSH

I went to Robert Creighton's farewell party. It was very good. I knew nearly everyone there. I wish Robert hadn't left. I got on well with him

Saw Dan. He was feeling very depressed. Who can blame him. In the evening he was sitting in a chair beside his bed. He is improving. I got him various soft drinks that he likes, and tintacks (a sweet he likes). He is now in RBC Ward.

Alison (Fundraising) gave me two lovely animal books for Yasmin, so I took them to her. Maureen (Alex Sister) came in, told me to sit down, and she put Yasmin in my lap so that I could read to her, which I did. Yasmin has an infection, so I have to put on an apron to see her.

Riza (Dialysis) was sitting near the front desk so we had a chat. She's great fun.

I wore the tie Shabnam sent me for Christmas. It has Happy Christmas and New Year in red and green narrow stripes all the way down, and a lot of people remarked on how attractive it is. Also, if you press a little button at the bottom of the tie it plays musical tunes; so when I went round the wards the children wanted to hear it. Jacob (L), 5, in Parrot Ward said he wanted to hear the singing tie.

I met a new family from Yugoslavia in Fox. Milaelo (J), 1+, has leukaemia. The family live here. Gordana, Mum, speaks excellent English.

I saw Lydia (C). She wasn't too well but, as I explained to her parents, the treatment does have lots of ups and downs, but it does so often provide the cure.

I also saw Christopher (M), 15 who has a heart and lung condition, and Wilma, his Mum who looked a little less depressed than before.

Rita was on duty in the Italian, so we had a long chat. If my next diary, Volume Four, comes in on time, I'll post a copy to her in America, where she is going for Christmas. She wants it out there, if possible.

Friday December 15, Dolphin Square

Good news today. Hammersmith Library have ordered, through their Leeds wholesaler, two of my diaries. If I could get the diaries into libraries it would be very encouraging. I found a note in my in-tray from Michelle (N). She is a lovely girl, 15, and has been through so much with renal problems, but is always happy and smiling. Very courageous. She often leaves me a note. We are great friends.

Saturday December 16, Dolphin Square

I'm working on my Christmas letters this weekend.

Sunday December 17, Dolphin Square

At the moment I've had to put everything on hold to get the Christmas letters out. I'll be glad when Christmas is over. I find it a very trying time of the year.

Monday December 18, Dolphin Square

Went to Leon Greenman's 90th birthday party this evening. It was held in a church hall near Euston station, so it was easy to get to, but I got soaked. An official sent me to the wrong side of the station, I hadn't brought an umbrella as it wasn't raining when I left, then it came down in buckets. My raincoat was soaked, and the top of my jacket. I had to dry out at the reception. Leon is remarkable. He was in five German concentration camps, principally Auschwitz, and he has an indomitable spirit. He has a remarkably strong will and outlook, especially considering all he's been through, having lost his wife and child who were gassed at Auschwitz. We have become good friends and I'm honoured to have his friendship. We write to each other regularly and he still types his own letters to his many friends and admirers.

I couldn't help reflecting, when the national Anti-Nazi leader got up to speak. She is a young Scots woman with a very broad accent. She ranted and raved, going on and on and on about the Nazis, and in this respect she was a female Goebbels whom I had seen, similarly ranting and raving in a TV programme on him the evening before. It is a gift. Goebbels brainwashed millions of Germans, this deformed little man with the power of oratory, and I could feel this with the Scottish woman, when the power of her oratory began to be convincing. Very dangerous.

Two very nice members of the Anti-Nazi League (they gave the party for Leon), Paul Honborow, with his wife Jan, gave me a lift back as they were passing here to go to their own home. I met there also another member I have known from past birthday parties for Leon, Cathy Hurrell, who is a teacher. Although she is in her late thirties, she has just become engaged to someone a little younger. She also is very nice and I like her a lot. I gave her advice on her wedding reception, telling her, among other things, to have a buffet, rather than a sit-down meal. I don't know if she will take my advice!

Tuesday December 19, GOSH

Spent most of today writing and sending Christmas letters (instead of cards), so far 129, and I have quite a few more to send. I went into GOSH late this afternoon, mostly for Nigel Clark's farewell party. He has done a magnificent job in charge of Fundraising, increasing the amount previously raised by £2,000,000 this year. He is a tall handsome man with a very attractive personality. There were a lot of people I knew including William Harkness, who I had bumped into beforehand and had a chat to then.

Before the party I went to see little Yasmin in Alexandra, who is going home for Christmas. In RBC Ward I saw Christopher (M) who was looking better because he's been able to get some sleep. He was just about to have his ankles (or near there) pierced to let out fluid. His legs are still very swollen but are going down. Then I saw Dan also in RBC. He was sitting in a wheelchair and was about to be taken up to see Mary (I don't know who she is) in DJW; but while I was there he was bending over and holding his head, and said he felt tired. I am very worried about him.

Going back to Nigel's reception, I had to leave at 7.00pm by taxi to go to Tim's organ recital at St Michael's, Cornhill, given in aid of GOSH. He is a brilliant player and I had a long talk to him afterwards. He was in GOSH for about ten years on and off, but I don't know what was wrong.

At GOSH I bumped into Dominic's (K) mother. Dominic had come in for emergency treatment as he was taken suddenly ill: he has cystic fibrosis. I didn't know he was there when I went to see Yasmin. Also in Alexandra I saw Sam (W) and gave him some money to go to the sweet shop. He is having an operation tomorrow. I'm not sure what he's in for. Alexandra is respiratory problems.

Wednesday December 20, Dolphin Square

I've found out what was wrong with Tim. It is printed in his organ recital programme. Among other things he was found to have gross food and chemical allergies and intolerances. He also has Asperger's Syndrome, the high achieving autism. GOSH had done a wonderful job. You wouldn't have known there is anything wrong with him. In the programme he said that without GOSH he would never have been able to achieve what he has done so far.

Thursday December 21, GOSH

Noel drove me, and Elaine, a Nurse in Churchill Day Care who looked after Scott, to Hitchin (Holwell) for Scott's funeral. The church was packed. He was buried in the church ground on this dry but cold day. We didn't go to the house but came straight back to GOSH.

I saw Yasmin and little Ben in Alexandra, then saw Aleema in Transitional Care, who was in bed with a mouth infection. I saw Sam (W) in PICU; he'd had his operation yesterday. He was sleepy so didn't talk much but is going back to Alexandra this evening. I also saw Christopher in RBC. He looked a little better; he's had his ankles pierced but said he was tired. I also saw baby Noah in CICU who'd had an operation to change his bowels over - they were twisted. He's come through it.

I had an early supper, chicken stir-fry, which was very nice. Afterwards I had a long chat to Inga in the Italian. She looked tired but it is always nice talking to her.

Friday December 22, Dolphin Square

Ronnie Page telephoned and I went down to see him. He gave me £75 for GOSH. He'd auctioned a squash racket that he's been given by the makers, and he added a cheque for £10 from himself. He does so much for the hospital.

I've been working again on Christmas letters and have cleared up most of them.

Nettie rang to tell me the sad news that Chris Edwards had died. He's had liver cancer for some time and hadn't told anyone. I'll write to Betty. Chris had just celebrated his 80th birthday.

Saturday December 23, Dolphin Square

Have just written a note to Bill about starting sittings for my portrait for the New Year.

On TV news it said five people were killed when their aircraft came down immediately after taking off. They were intending to go to Palma for Christmas, and the sunshine. You just never know.

There was also a programme on Alan Clark. I knew him well at Oxford. I never took to him. He died of a brain tumour.

Had a long telephone chat to Brenda Walker-Munro, and shorter one with Hugh. Euan, Susie and the children are spending Christmas Day with them.

Sunday December 24, Dolphin Square

I've been putting Rhoda's alterations into Volume Seven of the diaries. I spoke to her yesterday. She was packing as she's leaving today, with her family, to spend Christmas in Madrid.

The people who were killed in the light aircraft yesterday were a family. A millionaire racing promoter called Brian (I didn't get his surname), his brother, his son and daughter and a girl friend of the family. An awful tragedy. It was at Blackbush Airport and they were going to Minorca (not Palma) for a sunshine holiday.

Spoke to Kieran Stapleton. He and Barry are in their London home: the rest of the family have gone to their Irish home. I wished Kieran and Barry a happy Christmas.

Bobby rang to wish me a happy Christmas. He was quite surprised I'd got to Volume Seven.

Monday December 25, GOSH

I went to the hospital. It was quiet but I saw quite a few children, especially in Fox where they had a lovely party going in the playroom with lots of food. Baby Noah in CICU has improved and had his eyes open. There is a long scar down his tiny tummy where he's had open-heart surgery.

In Alexandra I saw Sam who looked better than last time. All his family were with him. I saw other children I knew.

I walked to GOSH from here, which took me about fifty minutes. It is cold outside, but I didn't have to walk back as Charlie, the Staff Nurse in Alexandra, insisted on driving me back. Lucy, the Staff Nurse in Clarence, also offered to drive me.

I had a delicious turkey lunch in the canteen, saw Stephen (Catering Supervisor) there and enjoyed the day very much.

Tuesday December 26, Dolphin Square

I have mentioned before the help given to me in the past by Frank Jackson and Alan Neame with my writing. I have always been very grateful to both of them.

There are now two others I have to thank. Rhoda Milne who has proof-read all my books and given me such valuable help and advice; also Bill Richards, who was in publishing all his life, designed the cover for my diaries, and has guided me in the commecial field of publishing. Without Rhoda and Bill I would not have achieved all that I have.

Wednesday December 27, Dolphin Square

I caught the 9.40am to Wivenhoe. Martyn came to meet me and I had the most delicious lunch which Pauline cooked. I enjoyed it very much. They came with me to Wivenhoe station and I caught the 3.00pm, breaking my journey at Witham. James met me there, and when I got to Goat Lodge a big family lunch was just finishing. James gave me a beautiful silk dressing gown that Robert had brought back from China and given to Edwin. I can use it when going for my morning swim.
Had a late Christmas card from Christine (U).

Thursday December 28, GOSH

Just waiting for Andy and Jane as we are going out.
Went into GOSH this morning and found a note in my in-tray from Annette (M) to say James was in Alexandra Ward. I was going there anyway, as Kathy O'Grady (Marks - Pantheon) gave me a lovely cake to take to GOSH for the nurses. I saw James and he's quite bright. He's on a breathing machine, and Annette said it's the first day for some time he's regained consciousness. He was talking a little and kept putting his finger in my mouth, and I pretended to bite it, which I used to do and this would make him laugh a lot, so obviously he remembered this. (Sister) Maureen was in the ward. When I went again, just before leaving, the whole family were there: Robert, Heather and her school friend and neighbour, Cloe.
I had a nice lunch in the Peter Pan cafe and on the way out saw Emma sitting with David. She told me they had become engaged on Christmas Eve, but wouldn't be getting married for about two years as they wanted to save up.
I had another Whitaker order from a Derbyshire bookshop for Volume Two of my diaries. It's good as I don't do any advertising.
9.50pm. Just come back from going out with Andy, Jane, Gemma and Hayden. The Fish & Chip shop was closed, so we went to Victoria Plaza, where we have been often and had a pizza. It was a most enjoyable evening. Very cold out. Hayden is such a good baby, a beautiful little boy. He's four months old now.
On the way out we met Stuart Sampson.

Friday December 29, Dolphin Square

Had a delightful day with Ali, Anita and the children. Ali brought Eleanor and Toby to Marylebone for the train ride, and I met them there. We caught a train straight back as one had been delayed and was just about to start. When we got to Chalfont St Giles where Ali had left the car there was thick snow and it was frozen. I was glad to get to the house, which is a very nice one, standing by itself.

Ali gave me a small bottle of very special whisky, from the Scottish Malt Whisky Society. It is 106.4% volume compared to the average malt of 70% and 43% volume. Actually, except when I'm out I've stopped drinking but I'll keep it here. He also gave me a very nice dark blue jacket which fits me.

One amusing Christmas card from Ellen Bannach who, although she speaks very good English, wrote:

Best wishes and greeting for a moody xmas with good people and a happy 2001.

Saturday December 30, Dolphin Square

I found some letters today, written by a young doctor over thirty years ago. At that time I was doing insurance and Nigel Stewart, then in his twenties, recently married, asked me to arrange life insurance for him, which I did. He was working at Gloucester Royal Hospital.

Some time later he found himself in financial difficulties and wanted to surrender the policy and I told him he would lose heavily on it; I told him to try and keep it going which he did. Six months later I had a message from his wife Trixi:

Nigel set out to climb Mont Blanc with two friends. They were nearing the summit of the climb when a storm broke, with high wind and blizzard. Nigel and his friends have never been seen since. Search parties and helicopters were sent out, but absolutely no trace of them whatsoever could be found.

It doesn't compensate for Nigel's loss, but I am glad I'd persuaded him to keep his policy.

Sunday December 31, GOSH

Darren Agius	25.09.90 - 12.05.96
Penelope Aitchison	03.04.68 - 10.08.68
Michael Aram	07.05.88 - 02.07.00
Alice Binks	13.09.95 - 07.10.95
Laura Brady	14.07.82 - 14.07.97
Felicity Brush	02.03.85 - 23.10.98
Jake Carr	04.05.96 - 28.10.98
Matthew Challen	05.09.80 - 03.11.98
Stephen Coomber	30.05.85 - 16.11.96
Bradley Dellar	16.12.86 - 28.02.99
Sonja Eyres	25.04.79 - 21.08.80
Sarah Evers	07.03.82 - 12.10.98
Edward Geffen	08.02.92 - 03.10.00
Zak Gilbert	11.09.95 - 16.08.00
Vanessa Gladden	10.09.85 - 27.05.00
Christopher Gummer	12.01.88 - 18.07.00
Mara Guppy	07.07.98 - 22.06.00
Cathal Hayes	15.04.93 - 11.09.98
Michelle Jones	06.04.90 - 21.07.00
Jenny-Rose Lotter	25.03.87 - 21.03.99
Ruhi Julie Parvez	25.04.84 - 19.10.99
Noah Phillips	26.10.00 - 11.03.01
Ryan Powell	30.12.97 - 29.06.00
Gary Pridmore	23.09.83 - 14.08.98
Scott Reidy	03.10.86 - 12.12.00
Max Rousham	06.01.99 - 21.11.99
Christopher Smith	25.06.89 - 04.03.00
Rachel Stocks	16.05.84 - 26.05.97
Alfie Sturge	21.01.92 - 15.10.00
Daniella Ford Welman	07.07.94 - 22.06.99
James White	05.08.88 - 28.02.98
John Williams	13.05.31 - 07.11.35

Jill walked along with me. I spoke about the loss of a child, and Jill, who is GOSH assistant Chaplain, told me that she had lost her little son, David, aged 5, twenty-two years ago. She said she felt angry and asked God why he had done this but then, after a time, although her life changed completely and was never the same again, she learned to accept it. You learn acceptance but the loss never goes away.

Wards

Alice
Dermatology
Endocrine

Annie Zunz
Rheumatology
Arthritis

Badger (formerly Alexandra)
Respiratory
Cystic Fibrosis
Chronic Lung Disease

Churchill
Neurology Medical

Churchill D.C.
Neurology Day Care

Clarence
Orthopaedic

Dickens
Programmed Medical Investigation
Endocrine
Metabolic
Renal
Gastro

David Waterston
Cardiac High Dependency

Elephant Day Care
Haematology
Oncology

Fox
Haematology
Oncology

Frederick Still
Metabolic
Endocrine
Bowel Diabetes

Giraffe
Immunology
Infectious Diseases
Host Defence

Helena
Gastroenterology (Medicine)

Island Day Care
Surgery

Lion
Haematology
Oncology
Host Defence

Louise
Urology

Mildred Creek
Eating Disorders
Psychological

Nuffield AB & DC
Private Patients

Parrot
Neurosurgery

Peter Pan
Ear
Nose
Throat

161

Robin
Haematology
Oncology
Bone Marrow Transplant

Tiger
Plastic Surgery
Craniofacial

Transitional Care
Long-Term Assisted Ventilation

Victoria
Renal
Dialysis
Kidney Transplant

Woodland (formerly Hedgehog & Rabbit)
General Surgery

CICU
Cardiac Intensive Care

NICU
Neo-Natal Intensive Care

PICU
Intensive Care

Medical Reference

Achilles Tendon
The tendon that pulls up the back of the heel.

Allergy
A collection of conditions caused by inappropriate or exaggerated reactions of the immune system to a variety of substances.

ALL   AML
Acute lymphoblastic leukaemia and acute myelogenous leukaemia. Acute leukaemia is that in which the white blood cells produced in excess within the bone marrow are immature cells called blasts. The abnormal cells may be of two types: lymphoblasts (immature lymphocytes) in acute lymphoblastic leukaemia, and myeloblasts (immature forms of other types of white cell) in acute myeloblastic leukaemia. Various subtypes are recognised according to the nature of the abnormal cells.

Aneurism
Abnormal dilation (ballooning) of an artery caused by pressure of blood flowing through a weakened area.

Arthritis
Inflammation of a joint characterised by pain, swelling and stiffness.

Asperger's Syndrome
A rare abnormality of development, possibly related to autism, that is characterized by subtle abnormalities of social interactions, preoccupation with special interests (such as prehistoric monsters, cars, etc.), and, commonly, by abnormalities of personality such as a particularly idiosyncratic sense of humour.

Autism
A condition in which a child is unable to relate to people and situations, and may show obsessive resistance to any change.

Atrium
Either of the two (right and left) upper chambers of the heart.

Baclofen
A muscle-relaxant drug that blocks nerve activity in the spinal cord. Baclofen relieves muscle spasm and stiffness that has been caused by injury to the brain or spinal cord, by a stroke, or by neurological disorders such as multiple sclerosis. Baclofen does not cure the underlying disorder but often allows physiotherapy to be more effective and makes walking and performing tasks with the hands easier. To reduce the risk of adverse effects, such as drowsiness and muscle weakness, the dose of the drug is usually increased slowly under medical supervision until the desired effect is achieved.

Baclofen Pump
The intrathecal baclofen pump administers baclofen directly into the spinal fluids.

Biopsy
A diagnostic test in which tissue or cells are removed from the body for examination under the microscope. Biopsy is an accurate method of diagnosing many illnesses, including cancer.

Bone Marrow
The soft fatty tissue found in bone cavities; it may be red or yellow. Red bone marrow is a blood producing tissue present in all bones at birth. During the teens it is gradually replaced in some bones by less active yellow marrow. Red bone marrow is the factory for most of the blood cells - all of red cells and platelets and most of the white cells. The blood cells go through various stages of maturation in the red marrow before they are ready to be released into the circulation. Yellow marrow is composed mainly of connective tissue and fat. If the body needs to increase its rate of blood formation, some of the yellow marrow will be replaced by red. Sometimes marrow fails to produce sufficient numbers of normal blood cells, as occurs in aplastic anaemia or when marrow has been displaced by tumour cells. In other cases marrow may overproduce certain blood cells, as occurs in polycythaemia and leukaemia.

Bone Marrow Transplant
The technique of using normal bone marrow to replace malignant or defective marrow in a patient.

Caesarian Section
An operation to deliver a baby from the uterus through a vertical or horizontal incision in the abdomen.

Cannula
A plastic or metal tube with a smooth unsharpened tip for inserting into a blood vessel, lymphatic vessel, or body cavity in order to introduce or withdraw fluids.

164

Cardio
To do with the heart

Catheter
A tube used to drain or inject fluid, or to apply pressure to a vessel. Catheters are commonly used to drain urine from the bladder. Other types are used to sample blood from the heart or to inject dye into the blood vessels during X-ray screening. Catheters are also used to unblock or widen obstructed blood vessels or to control bleeding.

Cerebral Palsy
A general term for disorders of movement and posture resulting from damage to a child's developing brain in the later months of pregnancy, during birth, in the newborn period or in early childhood. These disorders are non-progressive, i.e. the disability does not increase with time. The degree of disability is highly variable, ranging from slight clumsiness of hand movement and gait to complete immobility. In more than 90% of cases the damage occurs before or at birth.

Chemotherapy
The treatment of infection or cancer by drugs that act selectively on the cause of the disorder. Infections are treated by antibiotic drugs. Anticancer drugs act either by destroying tumour cells or by stopping them from multiplying. Because anticancer drugs act on all rapidly dividing cells, not just tumour cells, they can cause serious side effects including loss of hair and mouth ulcers.

Coma
A state of unconsciousness and unresponsiveness distinguishable from sleep in that the person does not respond to external stimuli e.g. shouting or pinching or to internal stimuli e.g a full bladder. Coma results from disturbance or damage to areas of the brain involved in conscious activity or the maintenance of consciousness. The damage may be the result of a head injury, or of an abnormality such as a brain tumour.

Cranialfacial
To do with the head (cranium) and face. There are many cranialfacial syndromes - children with unusual-shaped skulls.

CT Scanning
A diagnostic technique in which the combined use of a computer and X-rays passed through the body at different angles produces clear cross-sectional images ('slices') of the tissue being examined. CT (computed tomography) scanning provides clearer and more detailed information than X-rays used by themselves. CT scanning also has the advantage of tending to minimize the amount of radiation exposure.

Cystic Fibrosis

An inherited disease, present from birth, characterized by a tendency to chronic lung infections and an inability to absorb fats and other nutrients from food. The main feature is secretion of viscid (sticky) mucus which is unable to lubricate and flow freely in the nose, throat, airways and intestines

Dermatology

The branch of medicine concerned with the skin and the disorders that affect it. Also included in this specialty are the hair and nails, together with their various disorders. Problems include everything from wrinkles, warts, and hair loss to acne, athlete's foot and skin cancer.

Diabetes

Insipidus: Excessive production of urine due to an inadequate supply of a hormone secreted by the pituitary gland.

Mellitus: Disease in which the blood sugar is raised, due to insufficient insulin. The urine, which may be copious, contains glucose.

Dialysis

A technique used to remove waste products from the blood, and excess fluid from the body as a treatment for kidney failure.

Diaphragm

Dome-shaped muscle which separates the cavity of the thorax from the abdominal cavity. When it contracts and flattens, air is drawn into the lungs; it is one of the muscles of respiration.

Diarrhoea

Increased fluidity, frequency, or volume of bowel movements, as compared to the usual pattern for a particular person. Diarrhoea itself is not a disorder but is a symptom of an underlying problem.

Eczema

An inflammation of the skin, usually causing itching and sometimes accompanied by scaling or blisters. Some forms of eczema are better known as dermatitis. Eczema is sometimes caused by an allergy, but often occurs for no known reason.

Endocrine Gland

A gland that secretes hormones directly into the blood stream rather than through a duct. Examples of endocrine glands include the thyroid gland, ovaries, and adrenal glands which release thyroxine, oestrogens and hydrocortisone, respectively. The endocrine glands in the body make up the endocrine system.

Endotoxin
A poison produced by certain bacteria but not released until after the bacteria die; until then the toxin remains in the bacterial cell wall. Released endotoxins cause fever. They also make the walls of capillaries more permeable, causing fluid to leak into the surrounding tissue, sometimes resulting in a serious drop in blood pressure, a condition called endotoxic shock.

Enzyme
A protein that regulates the rate of a chemical reaction in the body. There are thousands of enzymes, each with a different chemical structure. It is this structure that determines the specific reaction regulated by an enzyme. To function properly many enzymes need an additional component called a coenzyme which is often derived from a vitamin or mineral. Every cell in the body produces various enzymes: different sets of enzymes occur in different tissues, reflecting their specialised functions. For example, the pancreas produces the digestive enzymes lipase, protease, and amylase; among the numerous enzymes produced by the liver are some that metabolize drugs.

Epidermolysis Bullosa
A group of rare inherited conditions in which blisters appear on the skin after minor damage. The disorder has a wide range of severity, from a type in which blisters form on the feet in hot weather, to a form in which there is widespread blistering and scarring. The condition is caused by a genetic defect. No special treatment for the condition is available, although injury to the skin should be avoided and simple protective measures should be taken to prevent the rubbing of affected areas when blisters appear. The outlook varies from a gradual improvement in mild cases to progressive serious disease in the most severe cases. Parents of affected children should obtain genetic counselling so that the risks of later children being affected can be calculated.

Epilepsy
A tendency to recurrent seizures or temporary alteration in one or more brain functions.

Exocrine Gland
A gland that secretes substances through a duct on to the inner surface of an organ or on to the outer surface of the body. Examples include the salivary glands, which release saliva into the mouth, the sweat glands, and the lacrimal glands which release tears. The release of exocrine secretions can be triggered by a hormone or by a neurotransmitter.

Exotoxin

A poison released by some types of bacteria into the bloodstream, from where it causes widespread effects throughout the body. Exotoxins are among the most poisonous substances known. They are produced by certain types of bacteria such as tetanus bacilli which enter the body through a wound and produce an exotoxin that affects the nervous system to cause muscle spasms and paralysis; and diphtheria bacilli which initially infect the throat but release an exotoxin that damages the heart and nervous system. Infections by tetanus, diphtheria and some other bacteria that release life-threatening exotoxins can be prevented by immunization with vaccines consisting of detoxified exotoxins.

Gastroenterology

The study of the digestive system and the diseases and disorders affecting it. The major organs involved include the mouth, oesophagus, stomach, duodenum, small intestine, colon and rectum. Diseases of the liver, gall-bladder and pancreas are also included in this specialty.

Gastroscopy

Examination of the lining of the oesophagus, stomach and duodenum (first part of the small intestine) by means of the endoscope, a long flexible viewing instrument called a gastroscope or oesophagogastroduodenoscope, inserted through the mouth. Gastroscopy is used to investigate symptoms such as severe pain in the upper abdomen or bleeding from the upper gastrointestinal tract, and to look for disorders of the oesophagus, stomach and duodenum.

Haematology

The study of blood and its formation, and the investigation and treatment of disorders affecting the blood and the bone marrow. Microscopic examination and counting of blood and bone marrow cells are essential procedures in diagnosing disorders such as anaemia and leukaemia.

Haemorrhage

The medical term for bleeding.

Hickman Line

Goes directly into the atrium (heart). Used for patients who are on long term 1V meds-treatment. Can also take blood from it. It is more comfortable than having cannulas and prevents having to use needles. It can be left in for long periods and patients can go home with it.

Hodgkins Disease

Also known as Hodgkin's lymphoma, a malignant disorder in which there is proliferation of cells in the lymphoid tissue (found mainly in the lymph nodes and spleen) and a resultant enlargement of the lymph nodes. Lymphoid tissue is an important part of the immune system. The cause of Hodgkin's disease is unknown.

Host Defence
Host defence encompasses haematology, oncology, immunology and bone marrow transplant; it assists the body's defence system against disease due to the body's inability to defend itself.

Hydrocephalus
An excessive amount of cerebrospinal fluid, usually under increased pressure within the skull. The term 'water on the brain' is a nonmedical phrase which is sometimes used to describe the condition. Hydrocephalus is often associated with other congenital abnormalities, particularly spina bifida.

Hydrocortisone
A corticosteroid drug used in creams, sprays and other topical preparations for the treatment of inflammatory or allergic conditions, such as ulcerative colitis or dermatitis. Hydrocortisone, also called cortisol, is a hormone produced by the adrenal gland.

Hypercalcaemia
An abnormally high level of calcium in the blood. Minor degrees of hypercalcaemia are quite common in healthy people and probably not significant. Hypercalcaemia is commonly caused by hyperparathyroidism, overproduction of parathyroid hormone, which helps control the blood calcium level. Less commonly it is due to excessive intake of vitamin D, which helps regulate the absorption of calcium, or to certain inflammatory disorders such as sarcoidosis.

Hyperlipidaemias
A group of metabolic disorders characterized by high levels of lipids (fats) in the blood.

Hypospadias
A congenital defect of the penis, occurring in about one in 300 male babies, in which the opening of the urethra is situated on the underside of the penis. The urethral opening may be on the glands (head) or shaft of the penis. In some cases the penis curves downwards, a condition known as chordee, and the foreskin is limited to the front of the penis. In severe forms of hypospadias the urethral opening lies well back along the penis towards the scrotum. The scrotum may be small, and the testes are undescended. In such cases the true sex of the child may be in doubt. Hypospadias can be corrected by a single operation in which the penis is straightened and a tube of skin (or occasionally bladder lining) is used to create a new urethra

169

that extends to the tip of the penis. The operation is normally performed before the child is two years old; circumcision should not be performed prior to a hypospadias repair because the foreskin may be needed at the operation. Surgery is usually successful, allowing the child to pass urine normally and, in later years, to have satisfactory sexual intercourse.

Immune System
A collection of cells and proteins that works to protect the body from potential harmful infectious microorganisms (microscopic life-forms) such as bacteria, viruses and fungi. The immune system also plays a role in the control of cancer, and is responsible for the phenomena of allergy, hypersensitivity, and rejection problems after transplant surgery.

Immunology
The discipline concerned with the immune system. Specialists in immunology are concerned with finding ways in which the immune system can be stimulated to provide immunity, principally through the use of vaccines. Immunologists also play an important part in transplant surgery, looking pre-operatively for a good immunological match between recipient and donor organ, and suppressing the recipient's immune system after transplantation to minimize the chances of organ rejection.

Intensive Care
The constant close monitoring of seriously ill patients, which enables immediate treatment to be given if the patient's condition deteriorates. The intensive care unit of a hospital contains electronic monitoring equipment that allows continuous assessment of vital body functions, such as blood pressure and heart and respiratory rates. The urine output, fluid balance, and blood chemistry of patients in intensive care units are recorded regularly. Medical and nursing staff are in a high ratio to patients and are specially trained in the techniques of resuscitation.

Intravenous Infusion
The slow introduction of a volume of fluid into the bloodstream. The fluid passes down from a plastic or glass container through tubing into a cannula (thin plastic tube) inserted into the vein, usually in the patient's forearm. The rate at which the fluid drips into the circulation is controlled by an adjustable valve.

Kawasaki Disease
An acute childhood illness that affects many systems in the body. It is also called mucocutaneous lymph node syndrome. The condition was first observed in Japan in the 1960s. It is becoming increasingly common in western countries. Kawasaki disease usually occurs in the first two years of life. The cause is unknown.

Leucotomy
The surgical operation of cutting some of the nerve fibres in the frontal lobes of the brain for treating intractable mental disorders.

Leukaemia
Any of several types of cancer in which there exists disorganized proliferation of white blood cells in the bone marrow (the tissue from which all blood cells originate). The reproduction of red blood cells, platelets, and normal white blood cells is impaired as normal cells are crowded out from the marrow by the leukaemia cells (abnormal white cells).

Life Support
The process of keeping a person alive by artificially inflating the lungs and, if necessary, maintaining the heartbeat with a pacemaker.

Lymphoma
Any of a group of cancers in which the cells of lymphoid tissue (found mainly in the lymph nodes and spleen) multiply unchecked. Lymphomas fall into two categories. If characteristic abnormal cells (Reed-Sternberg cells) are present, the disease is known as Hodgkin's lymphoma. All other types are called non-Hodgkin's lymphoma.

Meningitis
Inflammation of the meninges (the membranes that cover the brain and spinal cord) that usually results from infection by any of various microorganisms, usually a virus or a bacterium. Viral meningitis is relatively mild, but bacterial meningitis is life-threatening and requires prompt treatment.

Metabolic Disorders
A group of disorders in which some aspect of the body's internal chemistry is disturbed. Some metabolic disorders result from inherited abnormalities when a specific enzyme (a substance that promotes metabolic reaction) is absent or deficient or malfunctions in some way. Other metabolic disorders result from disorders of the endocrine system in which there is underproduction or overproduction of a hormone that controls metabolic activity. Examples include diabetes mellitus, Cushing's syndrome, insulinoma, hypothyroidism (underactivity of the thyroid gland) and hyperthyroidism ((overactivity of the thyroid gland). Other examples of metabolic disorders are porphyria, hyperlipidaemia, hypercalcaemia, gout and metabolic bone diseases such as osteoporosis, osteomalacia, rickets and Paget's disease.

Migraine
A severe headache, lasting anything from two hours to two days accompanied by disturbances of vision and/or nausea and vomiting. A

sufferer may experience only a single attack; more commonly, he or she has recurrent attacks at varying intervals.

MRI
Magnetic resonance imaging. MRI is a diagnostic technique that provides high quality cross-sectional or three-dimensional images of organs and structures within the body without using X-rays or radiation. Images from MRI are similar in many ways to those produced by CT scanning, but MRI generally gives much greater contrast between normal and abnormal tissues. MRI provides clear images of tumours of the brain and spinal cord. Also shown clearly by MRI is the internal structure of the eye and ear. MRI also produces detailed images of the heart and major blood vessels, provides images of blood flow, and is useful for examining joints and soft tissues, particularly in the knee.

Muscular Dystrophy
An inherited muscle disorder of unknown cause in which there is slow but progressive degeneration of muscle fibres. Different forms of muscular dystrophy are classified according to the age at which the symptoms appear, the rate at which the disease progresses, and the way in which it is inherited.

Neonate
A newly born infant under the age of one month.

Neurology
The medical discipline concerned with the study of the nervous system and its disorders, particularly with their diagnosis and treatment. Neurologists are trained to examine the nerves, reflexes, motor and sensory functions, and muscles to determine a disorder's cause and extent. To aid diagnosis, extensive use is made of modern imaging techniques such as CT scanning and MRI.

Neurosurgery
The specialty concerned with the surgical treatment of disorders of the brain, spinal cord, or other parts of the nervous system. Neurosurgery can deal with most conditions in which a localized structural change interferes with nerve function. Conditions treated by neurosurgery include tumours of the brain, spinal cord or meninges (membranes that surround the brain and spinal cord), certain abnormalities of the blood vessels that supply the brain, such as aneury (balloon-like swelling at a weak point in an artery), bleeding inside the skull, brain abscess, some birth defects such as hydrocephalus and spina bifida, certain types of epilepsy, and nerve damage caused by illness or accidents. Neurosurgeons are also concerned with the surgical relief of otherwise untreatable pain.

172

Node

A small rounded mass of tissue. The term most commonly refers to a lymph node, a normal structure in the lymphatic system.

Oesophagus

The muscular tube that carries food from the throat to the stomach. It acts as a conduit by which liquids and food are conveyed to the stomach and intestines for digestion. Food is propelled downwards towards the stomach by peristalsis (powerful waves of contractions passing through the muscles in the oseophageal wall). Gravity plays little part in getting food into the stomach, making it possible to drink while upside down.

Oncology

The study of the causes, development, characteristics, and treatment of tumours, particularly cancers (malignant tumours). Because there are many different types of tumours, deriving from virtually any tissue in the body, oncology encompasses a range of experimental techniques and investigative approaches. Doctors specialising in the study and treatment of cancer are known as oncologists. They are concerned with diagnosing the type of cancer and determining its exact location and rate of spread.

Orthopaedics

The branch of surgery concerned with disorders of the bones and joints and their associated muscles, tendons and ligaments. Orthopaedic surgeons perform many tasks, including setting broken bones and putting on casts; treating joint conditions such as dislocations, slipped discs, arthritis and back problems; treating bone tumours and birth defects of the skeleton; and surgically repairing or replacing hip, knee or finger joints.

Osteoblasts & Osteoclasts

The growth of bone is a balance between the activity of its two constituent cells, osteoblasts and osteoclasts. Osteoblasts encourage deposition of the mineral calcium phosphate in the protein framework of the bone. Osteoclasts remove mineral from the bone. The actions of these cells are controlled by hormones. These hormones also maintain the calcium level in the blood within close limits; any fall below the normal range affects the nerves and muscles.

Osteomalacia

Softening, weakening, and demineralization of the bones in adults due to vitamin D deficiency. In children the condition is called rickets. The development of healthy bone requires an adequate intake of calcium and phosphorous from the diet, but these minerals cannot be absorbed by the body without a sufficient amount of vitamin D. This vitamin is obtained from certain foods and from the action of sunlight on the skin; a deficiency results in softening and weakening of the bones, which then become vulnerable to distortion and fractures.

Osteomyelitis
Infection of bone and bone marrow, usually by bacteria. Osteomyelitis can affect any bone in the body, is more common in children, and most often affects the long bones of the arms and legs and vertebrae.

Osteopetrosis
A very rare inherited disorder in which bones harden and become more dense. The growth of healthy bone is a balance between the activity of two types of bone cells: bone-forming osteoblasts and bone-reabsorbing osteoclasts. In osteopetrosis there is a deficiency of osteoclasts, which results in the disruption of normal bone structure. More severe forms of osteopetrosis can result in greater susceptibility to fractures, stunted growth, deformity and anaemia. Pressure on nerves may cause blindness, deafness and paralysis.

Paediatrics
The branch of medicine concerned with the growth and development of children, and with the diagnosis, treatment and prevention of childhood diseases.

Paget's Disease
Paget's disease usually involves only limited areas. The normal process of bone formation is disrupted, causing the affected bones to weaken, thicken and become deformed. The bones usually affected are the pelvis, skull, clavicle (collarbone). vertebrae and long bones of the leg.

Pancreas
An elongated, tapered gland that lies across the back of the abdomen, behind the stomach. The broadest part of the pancreas (called the head) is situated on the right-hand side, in the loop of the duodenum. The main part of the gland (called the body) tapers from the head, extending towards the left and slightly upwards; the narrower end (called the tail) terminates near the spleen. Most of the pancreas consists of exocrine tissue, embedded in which are nests of endocrine cells (the islets of Langerhans). The exocrine cells secrete digestive enzymes into a network of ducts that meet to form the main pancreatic duct. This duct joins the common bile duct (which carries the gall bladder) to form a small chamber called the ampulla of Vater, which opens into the duodenum. The islets of Langerhans are surrounded by many blood vessels into which they secrete hormones. The pancreas has two functions: digestive and hormonal. The exocrine tissue secretes various digestive enzymes that break down carbohydrates, fats, proteins and nucleic acids. Most of these enzymes are inactive until activated in the

duodenum by other enzymes. Also secreted is sodium bicarbonate, which neutralizes stomach acid entering the duodenum. The endocrine cells in the islets of Langerhans secrete the hormones insulin and glucagon, which regulate the level of glucose in the blood.

Physiotherapy
Treatment of disorders or injuries with physical methods or agents. Physiotherapy is used to prevent or reduce joint stiffness and to restore muscle strength in the treatment of arthritis after a fracture has healed. It is also used to reduce pain, inflammation, and muscle spasm and to retrain joints and muscles after stroke or nerve injury. Physiotherapy is also concerned with the maintenance of breathing capacity in people with impaired lung function or the prevention and treatment of pulmonary complications following surgery. Physiotherapists help treat severe respiratory diseases (such as chronic bronchitis) and care for the respiratory needs of patients who are on ventilators or recovering from major operations.

Plastic Surgery
Any operation carried out to repair or construct skin and underlying tissue that has been damaged or lost by injury or disease, has been malformed since birth, or has changed with aging. Every attempt is made to maintain function of the affected part of the body and to create as natural appearance as possible. Operations performed mainly to improve appearance in an otherwise generally healthy person are known as cosmetic surgery. Plastic surgery is usually performed to repair damage caused by severe burns or injuries, and cancer. Among the congenital conditions that may require correction by plastic surgery are cleft lip and palate, hypospadias and imperforate anus. A variety of techniques is used to provide skin cover for damaged areas, including skin grafts, skin flaps, Z-plasty, and tissue expansion (in which skin is stretched by inserting a silicone balloon beneath the surface which is then gradually increased in size). These techniques may be combined with a bone graft or implants to provide underlying support. The scope of plastic surgery has been much broadened by the use of microsurgical techniques to join blood vessels, allowing the transfer of blocks of skin and muscle from one part of the body to another.

Platelet
The smallest type of blood cell, also called a thrombocyte. Platelets play a major role in blood clotting. A deficiency of platelets (a condition known as thrombocytopenia) can cause some types of bleeding disorders.

Polyarteritis Nodosa
An uncommon disease of medium-sized arteries, also called periarteritis nodosa. Areas of arterial wall become inflamed, weakened, and liable to

175

the formation of aneurysms (ballooned-out segments). Many different groups of blood vessels may be involved, including the coronary arteries that supply blood to the heart muscle, or the arteries of the kidneys, intestine, skeletal muscles, and nervous system. The seriousness of the condition depends on which organs are affected and how severely they are affected. The disease seems to be the result of a disturbance of the immune system (body's defences against infection), triggered in some cases by exposure to the hepatitis B virus.

Polycythaemia

A condition characterized by an unusually large number of red cells in the blood due to increased production by the bone marrow. This condition usually results from some other disorder or is a natural response to hypoxia (reduced oxygen in the blood and tissues). In such cases it is called secondary polycythaemia.

Porphyria

Any of a group of uncommon and usually inherited disorders caused by the accumulation in the body of substances called porphyrins. Sufferers often have a rash or skin blistering brought on by sunlight and may have abdominal pain and nervous system disturbances from certain drugs. Porphyrins are chemicals with a complex structure that are formed in the body during the manufacture of haem - a component of haemoglobin (the oxygen-carrying pigment in the blood).

Psychology

The scientific study of mental processes. Psychology deals with all internal aspects of the mind, such as memory, feelings, thought and perception, as well as external manifestations such as speech and behaviour. Psychology is also concerned with intelligence, learning and personality development. Within psychology a number of different approaches are used. Neuropsychology attempts to relate human behaviour to brain and body functions. Behavioural psychology studies the ways in which people react to events and learn to adapt accordingly. Cognitive psychology concentrates on thought processes, and is based on the theory that what a person thinks about his or her behaviour is of equal importance to the behaviour itself. Psychoanalytic psychology stresses the role of the unconscious and of childhood experiences. There are many specialised areas within the science. Educational psychologists study learning and intelligence; clinical psychologists are concerned with emotional and behavioural problems; social and industrial psychologists consider the effects of work and the environment on behaviour; and experimental psychologists concentrate on research into new ways of understanding mental events. The emergence of development psychology as a specialist area is due to the work of the Swiss psychologist Jean Piaget, who noted that a child's intellectual development passes through certain stages -from simple motor skills to logical and abstract thought.

Pulmonary
Pertaining to the lungs. For example, the pulmonary artery is the blood vessel that carries blood from the heart to the lungs.

Radiotherapy
Treatment of cancer, and occasionally other diseases, by X-rays and other sources of radioactivity. Sources of this kind produce ironizing radiation which, as it passes through the diseased tissue, destroys or slows down the development of abnormal cells. Provided the correct dosage of radiation is given, normal cells suffer little or no long-term damage. Transient side-effects that develop during treatment are, however, a reflection of acute damage to normal tissue. Radiotherapy is often used after surgical excision of a malignant tumour to destroy any remaining tumour cells.

Reflux
An abnormal backflow of fluid in a body passage due to failure of the passage's exit to close fully. The most common types of reflux are regurgitation of acid fluid from the stomach into the oesophagus, and the backflow of urine from the bladder into one or both ureters (ves-ico-ureteric reflux). Persistent reflux of urine may lead to kidney damage.

Renal
A medical term meaning related to the kidney.

Respiration
A term for the process by which oxygen reaches body cells and is utilized by them in metabolism, and by which carbon dioxide is eliminated.

Rhabdomyosarcoma
A very rare, malignant tumour of muscle. Rhabdomyosarcoma may develop during infancy, usually affecting the throat, bladder, prostate gland or vagina. The tumour grows rapidly and spreads to other tissues. Treatment is by surgical removal, combined with radiotherapy and anticancer drugs.

Rheumatology
The branch of medicine concerned with the causes, development, diagnosis and treatment of diseases that affect the joints, muscles, and connective tissue. Rheumatologists use a variety of investigative techniques, ranging from X-rays of joints to tests of muscle function and blood analysis. Treatment is similarly varied, including drug treatment with anti-inflammatory drugs or analgesic drugs, and physiotherapy.

Sarcoidosis

A rare disease of unknown cause in which there is inflammation of tissues throughout the body, especially in the lymph nodes, lungs, skin, eyes and liver. The disorder occurs mainly in young adults.

Scrotum

The pouch that hangs behind the penis and contains the testes. The scrotum consists of an outer layer of thin, wrinkled skin over a layer of muscle-containing tissue.

Sebaceous Glands

Minute glands in the skin that secrete a lubricating substance called sebum. Sebaceous glands either open into hair follicles or discharge directly on to the surface of the skin. They are most numerous on the scalp, face and anus; they do not occur on the palms of the hands or the soles of the feet. The production of sebum by the sebacious glands is partly controlled by androgen hormones (male sex hormones).

Shunt

An abnormal or surgically created passage between two normally unconnected parts. The term shunt is usually used to refer to a passage created to relieve abnormal fluid pressure around the brain in hydrocephalus or to relieve pressure in the portal veins in portal hypertension. The shunt for hydrocephalus consists of two catheters and a valve to prevent backflow. The first catheter is inserted through the skull to drain fluid from the ventricles of the brain. The second is passed into another body cavity, usually the abdominal cavity or the right atrium of the heart, where the excess fluid is absorbed. Various surgical procedures may be used to reduce pressure in the portal system (the veins that carry blood from the digestive organs and spleen to the liver) and so reduce the risk of bleeding.

Spina Bifida

A congenital defect in which part of one or more vertebrae fails to develop completely, leaving a portion of the spinal cord exposed. Spina bifida can occur anywhere on the spine but is most common in the lower back. The severity of the condition depends on how much nerve tissue is exposed. The cause of spina bifida remains unknown; it is thought that many factors are involved.

Staphylococcal Infections

A group of infections caused by bacteria of the staphylococcus genus. Staphylococci, which grow in grape-like clusters, are a common cause of skin infections but can also cause serious internal disorders. Staphylococcal bacteria are present harmlessly on the skin of most people. If the bacteria become trapped within the skin by a blocked

178

sweat or sebaceous gland, they may cause superficial skin infections such as pustules, boils, abscesses, styes or carbuncles. Infection of deeper tissues may result if the skin is broken. Staphylococcal bacteria are also harmlessly present in the membranes that line the nose and throat. In newborn babies, toxins released by bacteria on the skin can cause a severe blistering rash called the scalded skin syndrome.

Steroid Drugs
A group of drugs that includes the corticosteroid drugs, which resemble hormones produced by the cortex adrenal glands, and the anabolic steroid drugs. Anabolic steroids, by mimicking the anabolic effects of testosterone, build tissue, promote muscle recovery following injury, and help strengthen bones. They are given to treat some types of anaemia. Anabolic steroids have been widely abused by athletes who wish to improve their strength and stamina. This practice has serious risks to health.

Stroke
Damage to part of the brain caused by interruption to its blood supply, or by leakage of blood through the walls of blood vessels. Sensation, movement, or function controlled by the damaged area is impaired. Certain factors increase the risk of having a stroke. The two most important are hypertension (high blood pressure) which weakens the walls of the arteries, and atherosclerosis (narrowing of arteries by fatty deposits).

Testis
One of two male sex organs, also called testicles, that produce sperm and the male sex hormone testosterone.

Thyroxine
The most important thyroid hormone produced by the thyroid gland.

Toxin
A poisonous protein produced by pathogenic (disease-causing) bacteria such as clostridium tetani, which causes tetanus; various animals and reptiles, notably venomous snakes; or certain plants, such as the death cap mushroom Amanita Phaloides. Bacterial toxins are sometimes subdivided into three categories: endotoxins. which are released only from the inside of dead bacteria; exotoxins, which are released from the surface of live bacteria; and anterotoxins, which inflame the intestine.

Toxic Shock Syndrome
An uncommon severe illness caused by a toxin produced by the bacterium staphylococcus aureus. The onset of toxic shock syndrome is sudden, with high fever, vomiting, diarrhoea, headache, muscular aches and pains, dizziness and disorientation. A skin rash resembling sunburn develops on the palms and soles, and peels within one or two weeks. The

blood pressure may fall dangerously low, and shock may develop. Other serious complications include kidney failure and liver failure.

Tracheostomy
An operation in which an opening is made in the trachea (windpipe) and a tube is inserted to maintain an effective airway. Tracheostomy may be performed to treat an emergency or as a planned procedure. Today acute airway problems are usually handled by an endotracheal tube passed via the mouth or nose. A tracheostomy is preferable, however, for the emergency treatment of airway problems (such as a tumour or a foreign body) involving the larynx. A planned tracheostomy is most commonly performed on a person who has lost the ability to breathe naturally and is undergoing long-term ventilation (the pumping of air into the lungs by a machine) or who has lost the ability to keep saliva and other secretions out of the trachea because of coma, or a specific airway or swallowing problem. In such cases, tracheostomy is performed after passing an endotracheal tube through the nose or mouth and into the trachea. Permanent tracheostomy is necessary after laryngectomy (surgical removal of the larynx).

Urethra
The tube by which urine is secreted from the bladder. In females the urethra is short and opens to the outside just in front of the vagina between the labia minora. In males the urethra is much longer. It is surrounded by the prostate gland at its upper end and then forms a channel through the length of the penis.

Wilm's Tumour
A type of kidney cancer, also called nephroblastoma, that occurs mainly in children.

Z-plasty
A technique that is used in plastic surgery to change the direction of a scar so that it can be hidden in natural skin creases or to relieve skin tension caused by contracture of a scar. Z-plasty is especially useful for revising unsightly scars on the face and for releasing scarring across joints, such as on the fingers or in the armpits, that may restrict normal movement or cause deformity. A Z-shaped incision is made with the central arm of the Z along the scar. Two V-shaped flaps are created by cutting the skin away from underlying tissue. The flaps are then transposed and stitched. The procedure has the effect of redistributing tension perpendicular to the original defect.

Only illnesses and diseases suffered by the children recorded in this diary are given. Parents wrote them in my notebook alongside their children's names. About three could not be found, either because the parent had got it wrong or had completely misspelt, excusable when dealing with medical terminology.

Short History of the Hospital

On St. Valentine's Day, 14 February 1852, the country's first hospital for sick children opened its doors in Great Ormond Street with ten beds. It was the inspiration of Dr Charles West who, appalled by the lack of facilities for very ill children in the capital, had set about raising money for the cause.

The new Hospital attracted public support. Queen Victoria, Charles Dickens and J.M Barrie, who donated to the Hospital copyright of his famous play Peter Pan, were among those to pledge their help.

The Hospital grew and developed. In 1893 a new purpose built wing was opened with room for 240 beds and 15 years later, a whole new outpatients department was built with funding from Mr William Astor.

After the Second World War, the Institute of Child Health opened and began its pioneering research into discovering cures and developing treatments for children's illnesses in conjunction with Great Ormond Street Children's Hospital. Building work, modernising and updating parts of the hospital continued throughout the years establishing Great Ormond Street as one of the leading children's hospitals in the world.

The Institute of Child Health is in a separate building but works in partnership with GOSH. It is the largest paediatric research, teaching and training centre in Britain. Researchers pool their efforts, tackling issues to improve child health. The research is based on these themes:

Cancer
Cardiospiratory Sciences and Vascular Biology
Interrelated Disease and Congenital Malformations
Infection and Immunity
Nutrition
Population Health Sciences

Today TV coverage shows clearly to millions the care and devotion doctors, nurses and other members of staff give to sick children; in this respect Great Ormond Street is no different to other children's hospitals. What does make this hospital exceptional is the number of specialist surgeons and physicians who deal not only with children coming direct to GOSH, but also the large number of referrals from other children's hospitals throughout the country and abroad, children with rare and often life-threatening illnesses.

Consultants are attached to the ward dealing in their specialities; the structure of one ward is an illustration of how other wards work in this way.

Clarence is an orthopaedic ward, into which four surgeons admit their patients.

Mr Jones specialises in correcting Talipes (club feet) and dislocated hips in young children.

Mr Noordeen specialises on children with scoliosis and other spinal problems.

Mr Hill's main interest is limb lengthening using Ilizarov frames. These were first used in Russia for surgery on legs, but Mr Hill pioneered their use for lengthening the humerus (upper arm).

Mr Monsell specialises in complex repositioning of hips in older children to aid with seating.

The reason for referrals from other children's hospitals is that these surgeons have skills to carry out highly complex operations, nor available in the local hospital.

Many GOSH surgeons and physicians have international reputations usually only known in the medical world, but sometimes, because of the nature of their work, they become public figures such as Professor Spitz, who has separated conjoined twins. Many GOSH consultans are leaders in their own field, loved by their little patients and having the gratitude of families whose children's health is dependent on the consultant's skill.

In addition to the doctors, every ward has a dedicated team of Staff. On Clarence Ward this includes:

Lucy Howlett, Spinal Sister

Kerry Simpson, Ward Sister

Julia Lomax, Orthopaedic Case Manager (co-ordinating admissions & discharges).

As well as these three senior staff, the other nurses, junior doctors, play specialists and other members of the multi-disciplinary team. contribute to the high quality of care given to the patients.

184

*Thoughts on Great Ormond Street
by some of the Children*

Jack Kershaw

Born with a rare and chronic form of combined Immune Dificiency which was diagnosed when he was 3, Jack came to GOSH two years later for a Bone Marrow Transplant, his only hope of a cure. Four years later a suitable donor was found. The immediate results were a great success but sadly, not long after writing about GOSH, Jack lost his battle and died on 15 January. A brave boy, always cheerful, he was good company, and his concern for others can be seen in his poem, He is greatly missed, not only by his family, but by all who had the privilege of knowing him.

My name is Abigail Spencer. I am 2 years old. I have been coming to G.O.S.H. since I was born. I have only had a few weeks at home and live in hospital. I have lots of things wrong with me, but they don't stop me from smiling. 😁

I was born with Pierre Robin Syndrome, Cystic fibrosis and Autoimmune Enteropathy. I am also moderately deaf.

I don't mind it in hospital as it is home to me and I know all the Drs and nurses and have made lots of friends.

I have a lot of line + chest infections as I have a nasty bug in my lungs. I have lots of nubulizers to help me breathe better. I used to have a artificial airway for a year, but I don't need it anymore! Mummy has to do chest physiotherapy to clear my chest – It's really boring; so I watch the Tweenies. F133 is my favourite 🎵

I do not eat food as I can't swallow properly, but I like playing with plastic food. I have a hole in my tummy that I have my medicines in. Mummy says its called a "gastrostomy". I used to be really skinny, now I have a special food called TPN, which goes into a plastic tube into my chest (Huckman catheter) This has made me fatter. I get told off for playing with my pumps. I have to have lots of tests and bloods taken – Sometimes it hurts and Mummy gives me a sticker as I have been a brave girl. ⭐ The play specialist takes my mind off it by blowing bubbles °°₀ She also takes me down the play centre which is really good fun! Sometimes I get frustrated when I can't play properly as I am connected to my pumps for most of the day. The doctors and nurses are really nice, they help me feel better, they also have fun with me. I like music and dancing, so we all boogie together!

I don't go anywhere without my Zebra, he is my favourite toy and has lots of things done to him, the same as me. I love him to bits, he helps me not to cry and helps me sleep. Me and my Zebra like lots of cuddles

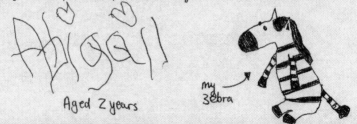

Abigail

Aged 2 years

my Zebra

Abigail Spencer, age 2

Harry Matthews-Hall   Age 5

I first went to Gosh when I was 4½ because my arm had stopped working and I had lost my smile. The Doctors couldn't find it anywhere.

My Mummy said that I have cancer and it is hiding in my brain and neck.

I've had lots of cannulars and they made me blow up a green balloon. It made me very sleepy and grumpy. Now I have wigglies. I have my medicine through them and that means no more cannulars or green balloons. I have chemotherapy and radiotherapy which makes my hair fall out. I am finding my smile again, I have kinks and my Mummy says I am hansome and very brave.   P.T.O.

Harry Matthews-Hall, age 5

I miss swimming and school but when
I have my wigglies out I can do all
my favourite things.
My special friend on Lion Ward is Jessie
she plays with me in the play room, and
paints pictures with me.

Harry Matthews-Hall

190

I first came to G OSH when I was baby. I have a problem with
my bones growing and now go every six months. I like going
because it does not feel like a hospital and everyone is my friend
Andrew Bastin----aged 6

I First came to GOSH when I wa a baby.
I have a problem with my bones
growing and now go every six months.
I like going because it dois not feel
like a hospital and everyone is my
friend

Andrew Bastin aged 6

Andrew Bastin, age 6

Charlie Wisdom   **Age 6**

I have leukaemia, and I have been in Great Ormond Street since April. I have chemo treatment and I was very unwell, but I now feel much better.
I like being in GOSH because it is better than being in our local hospital. I like it here because there is a playroom. I have a Play Specialist, Jessie, and I call her Messy Jessie because she's always mixed up with paints. My nurse, Louise, I call Loopy Lou because we have pretend fights, and she gets her own back by calling me Cheeky Charlie. I made friends with Brennan (Brennan Briggs 6) who is here with lymphoma, and Sam (Sam Stockwell 4) who is in Lion Ward having treatment.

I am on my last treatment and go home at the end of this week and will see my goldfish Peter III Wisdom. He is called this because I had two other goldfish who died, and I have called them all Peter. I like this Peter III because in the summer he has black patches and he goes all gold in the winter.

Charlie Wisdom, age 6

Thoughts on Great Ormond Street

When I first went to Great Ormond Street Hospital I was 7 months old. I had my first 'big' operation when I was 1.......it was very scary! The good thing about GOSH is that you meet lots of good friends. I do not like operations because they are very scary, the mask is horrible and it 'stinks'!

When I first started coming to GOSH I did not like the clowns because I was only young and they frightened me. Now when I meet the clowns, I make them laugh! I met William when I was 1; he is a very nice and kind man. Every time I'm in hospital he comes to see me. We talk about stuff like football and he gives me money for sweets.

So far I have had 14 operations and I might have to have some more. I have got a very poorly tummy and I've got a gastrostomy tube. My doctor is Dr. Lindley and he is a nice man who makes me laugh.

As I am getting older, I understand more about my operations and my illness and coming to GOSH isn't too bad (but I'd rather be playing football!)

Jack Bennett

Age 7 3/4

Jack Bennett, age 7

My name is Lauren Spelman I am ten years old.
When I was one year old I was diagnosed with a Brain Tumour.
I have had Radiotherapy and Lots of different chemo therapy
treatments.
I went to Elephant ward for my chemo. I met some nice nurses
there and Ski was my consultant.
Three years ago I had problems with my shunt and had to have
lots of operations. I had some of my tumour taken out too.
I was in and out of hospital for several months. I really liked it
on parrot ward and I have lots of friends there. I had a teacher called
Catherine from the hospital school who came to teach me every day.
I liked going to the play centre and I went to Brownies in the
hospital too.
My nurses Harry, Melissa, Amanda, and Lesley took me to see Britney
Spears in concert and I met ~~her~~ her before the show. It was very exciting
My tumour has not grown for a while and I feel great.
I still see Mr Harkness, my Neuro surgeon regularly.
I've had lots of good times at Great Ormond Street Hospital.

Lauren Spelman, age 10

194

This is a Poem I wrote before coming into hospital.

Now our countries are going to war,
It makes me reely want to roar,
Bombs that make places shatter,
While Tony blair and George w natter,
While the towers were bombed that was shocking,
But is the answer to send more bombs Dropping,
People like you and me who are frightend and scared
While those worried Afgalnistan families beware,
exsPolins that made those big buildings fall,
We wish they never happened at all,
Even though thousands died ... Its not right
that more innicint people Should die in this fight.

by Jack edward kershaw Age 10

Jack Kershaw, age 10

I came to Great ormand street In June for a Bone marrow Transaplant and I went home In September but I had to come back In November and I have been on Robin ward ever since. I was allowed to go home for Christmas for a few hours. I Like my school Teacher Anna and Play Specialist Rachel, she arranged for Arsenal to see me. Its hard being In my room but I am allowed to go to the gym. My favourite nurses are Cian, Helen, ceri, Tania, Lesley, chris. Mum stays with me and My brother, nanna and dad come up to see me. Its not very nice being In hospital and I miss all my friends at home in Tawcester. All the Docters are trying there best to make me better. I enjoy getting letters from school and other people. I think its funny when the clowns come up and see me. I am going to be 11 years old in January. Hopefully I will be able to go home and Play on My new Playstation 2.

Jack Kershaw

My name is Daniel Plenderleith and I am 10 years old I'v got Leukaemia. I was diagnosed with Leukaemia on Christmas eve 1998, it wasn't very nice spending Christmas in hospital because I couldn't open my presents without a bit of help from my mum or dad. Great Ormand street really looked after me, my consultant David webb is really nice. Great Ormand Street is one of the best hospitals I have ever been in. I like the playrooms they have lots of toys, theres always lots of fun things to do in the play-area's. While I was in hospital I made 3 friends so I wasn't on my own all the time

Daniel Plenderleith, age 10

Great Ormond Street **NHS**
Hospital for Children
NHS Trust

Great Ormond Street
London WC1N 3JH
Tel: 020 7405 9200

23rd July 2002

Dear William

I have been coming to GOSH for 9 months

I have just had a 5 and a 1/4 hour operation

To Remove my large colon Which has Been
ulceratied and bleeding. But Now it has
gone I feel much better. I am with mummy
and daddy and my Sister Lucia in
woodland ward hoping to go home
soon.

From
Charlie Traylen
age 10

In Partnership with the Institute of Child Health, UCL
Patron: Her Majesty The Queen
Chairman: Sir Cyril Chantler MA MD FRCP FRCPCH FMedSci

Charlie Traylen, age 10

Dear William,

Hope you are well. Since my operation in may I have been very well. I am very pleased with what the doctors have done.

I started my new school in September and like it although I get lots of homework now. We break up for our Christmas holiday this Friday for two weeks.

I wrote this poem at school,

In the town of Jerusalem Mary came home, she had the son of god.
But she was a virgin,
They travelled to Bethlehem, with a donkey with Mary on the back,
There was no room in the inn,
So they had Jesus in a stable, he was put in a manger,
kings came with gifts, gold frankincense and Muir,
Shepherds followed the star, they came to see the new born,
Ox, as and donkey watched over him.

On December 3rd I came to hospital to see Mr Ransley. They were very pleased.
We went to the shop and bought your book and I saw my name in it and my moms.
My brother read it on the way home on the train then we all read it. It was nice seeing my name in your book.

I am hoping to have a video machine for my bedroom and some music CDs for Christmas.
Have a nice Christmas,
Best Wishes,
 Stephen Grosvenor

Dear William,
        Since Stephen's op. in May he has been very well and the op. was a great success. We both have not forgot your kindness during his stays in hospital and Stephen always mentions your name when he talks of his hospital times. As Stephen mentions in his letter we all enjoyed your book and it gave us more of an insight into how much time you give to the parents and children. Your kindness is much appreciated.
        Stephen has no other major operations planned for a few years until he reaches puberty! Many out-patient check ups though, so I'm sure we will see you again soon.
        Best wishes for Christmas and New Year
                                    Julie & family.

Stephen Grosvenor, age 11

My name is: Laura Topliss

Age: 11

I've been coming to Great Ormond Street Hospital for 11 years. Its the best Hospital ever.

Problem: When i was 8 months old i had to have a new heart because i was born with cardiomyppathy and a heart block it was really bad. When i was 9 years old i had to have another heart because it had a disease around it and it could'nt pump Properly and it Failed. At first i said to my doctor that i did not want one because i might die. Then when i went home i wrote a letter and said i would like one to make me feel better but at the momment life is up and down. But the doctors and nurses are great.

Laura Topliss, age 11

MY EXPERIENCES AT GOSH

My name is Sian and I have a metabolic disease, which has also caused problems with my kidneys. I come to GOSH every two months for outpatients clinics and sometimes I have to stay, either because I am unwell or need tests. I usually stay on Frederick Still Ward.

For me, there are two really good things about staying at GOSH. The first is Radio GOSH. Last time I had to stay, Kate (my nurse) took me up to Radio GOSH. It was a bit of a struggle because we had to fit my wheelchair and a drip stand on to the lift but Peter from Radio GOSH helped us. I had a really good time and I talked on the radio. Next time I have to stay I'll definitely go back to Radio GOSH – it really cheered me up! The second thing I really like are the Clown Doctors. Before I came to GOSH I was looked after at Guy's Hospital and Dr Kiku and Dr Mattie used to come to see me there. When I came to GOSH they came to see me straight away and it was really nice to see somebody I already knew. The Clown Doctors always make me laugh. I have even called my rabbit after Dr Kiku!

20.01.2002

Dear William,

Thank you for coming to see Siân on Frederick Still ward last Tuesday. Siân had surgery to put in a new port-a-cath on Wednesday and was well enough to go home on Thursday evening.

As promised, Siân has written a piece about her experiences at G.O.S.H which you may wish to include in the new section of your diary. Siân decided not to give too much personal information about her disease, treatment and prognosis.

Good luck with the Diary - we will keep an eye open for it in the hospital shop - and thank you again for taking the time to visit Siân.

Best wishes

Sue Gorvett (Siân's mum)

Sian Gorvett, age 12

David Hewes   **Age 12**

I have been in GOSH many times in my life and have grown to like the atmosphere. I first went in when I was three and at the time I was very ill with cancer of the bladder. I don't remember very much about that period in my life. I only know that they must have done a pretty good job because I am here, and writing this now, aged 12!

Every child knows deep down that the Doctors and Nurses are only trying to help and hate it if you are frightened. I think they do an amazing job in persuading kids to accept all kinds of different and perhaps scary treatments. They also succeed in relaxing children before they undergo any medication.

I recently returned for constructive surgery and remembered how the Doctors and Nurses try to bribe the little ones with stickers, but I have now been upgraded to certificates! I will always recall the look of surprise on the porter's face as he wheeled me towards the theatre. I was so excited because the operation was such a step forward in my life.

When I was recovering a play specialist on Louise ward named Fiona came and helped me to get back on my feet, literally. Nearly every day she decided upon a new project that we could do together.

I realise that many people think that GOSH is a sad place. It is not. Of course there are sad cases but I will only look back on the good times, as there are many more of them.

David Hewes, age 12

Lion Ward

Great Ormond Street
Hospital for Children
NHS Trust

Great Ormond Street
London WC1N 3JH

Tel: 020 7405 9200

Dear William,

Very best wishes

For your diary

29.07.02

With lots of love

Jack Payne x+x

aged 12

P.S. Thank you for the sweeties!

In Partnership with the Institute of Child Health, UCL
Patron: Her Majesty The Queen
Chairman: Sir Cyril Chantler MA MD FRCP FRCPCH FMedSci

The child first and always

Jack Payne, age 12

I m Charlie Pleasants, I went to GOSH with a water weres problem if you get what I meen. Affter one day of beeing at GOSH I went into an operating thiater under genral anasthetic. When I came out out of the anasthetic I found out the had found a piece of tisue block-ing the ureathra and they had cut it away. When a nurs took out the cath alther I ded what you call a flowrate test which says how fast your peeing. before I had the oparation it took two minute until I finish weeing after the operation it took less than 5 seconds. All this treet ment hapne in three days of beeing at gosh. Before I went in to the operating theater I felt alitle bit frightend but afterworts when I fown out I was better it all payd off.

Charlie Pleasants, age 12

Dear William,

   I hope you are keeping well. Thank you for your last letter and the chance to write an article to go into your book. I would love to take the opportunity to do so. I have come up with a piece and it is as follows:

My name is Adam Keogh and I am thirteen years of age. In December 1989 when I was 18 months old I was referred to GOSH to see a doctor who specialised in spinal problems. I have scoliosis; which is curvature of the spine. We have seen the redevelopment and many alterations to the hospital over the years we have been coming, it is now a bright friendly place that is very well equipped to make your visit as easy as possible and I think it is the best children's hospital in the world.

The years I have been visiting the hospital have always seemed like a day out so when I was ten years of age and told I had to have an operation as my spine was rapidly getting worse I couldn't believe it was going to happen. I have always enjoyed playing lots of sports and this would change my life. On the 17th August '98 my family and I travelled down to London, that night we stayed in a travel lodge as the next day I was going into GOSH for two days of tests before the operation. I was very upset and didn't want to talk to anybody but I knew I had to have the operation done before it became even worse so I persevered. While I was waiting different people were coming to see me like the anaesthetist, surgeon, pain relief doctor, they were trying to explain what would happen and that I would have tubes in various places for different reasons. There were also other people who would visit like play specialist and clowns who would try to distracted you and help you to relax. William was visiting the ward when he spotted my Chelsea shirt; we would sit and talk about football, mainly Chelsea because we both support them. It was very strange on the ward because with it being orthopaedic most of the children were in bed and not able to move around. I found it very disturbing to see so many children suffering.

On the 20th august I spent the whole of the day in surgery, my parents were waiting for me and as soon as I was stabilised Lucy the spinal nurse took me back to the ward.

The following day was a big day for Lucy, she had a television crew following her around all day filming for This Morning who were doing a

Adam Keogh, age 13

career profile on nursing. As I was Lucy's patient I was filmed a little but was too poorly to take a lot of interest.

The days after the operation went really slowly and I was in a lot of pain. William called to see me on the Saturday, he had been to watch Chelsea and had called into the hospital with the programme for me, this brighten my day. One week after the operation I was fitted with a brace that protected my back and restricted my movements to prevent any damage. I had to wear this all the time for the next few months even to sleep in, at least I was able to get out of bed though.

My operation was three years ago and I am now playing most sports again and living a busy happy life. I am very grateful for what GOSH was able to do for me I still visit for checks and I like to keep in contact with William who keeps me up to date with the hospital news.

I hope this is something that you are looking for and I haven't made it too long. I have nearly finished the book, mum read it in two days and said it made her feel very sad for the children who are poorly and their families, but we think you are wonderful in the time and patience that you give to the children, especially when the circumstances are so difficult and upsetting. We were really sorry to read about your godson's accident and we hope you are remembering the happy times that you spent with him. I am putting a cheque in the envelope for the book and would like to say thank you for sending it to us. Maybe if there is another published with more in you will let us know. I have been home from school today because I have a sore throat and sickness bug, this evening I am feeling a little bit better and hopefully tomorrow I will be able to go to school again.

I would like to wish you a happy Christmas and will write again in the new year.

Adam
Keogh

Adam Keogh

206

Saturday 15th December

Dear William

Thank-you for remembering me. I would love to do an article for your book. Enclosed is a piece of writing about a stay I had in Dickens. I hope it is all right, and you can use it. I hope you are keeping well, and have a good Christmas.

Love from Stephi

My name is Stephi Reynolds; I am 13 years old and have Inflammatory Bowl Disease (IBD). I have been on Dickens Ward many times but strongly remember my first stay on there. I was 9, I had to have a lot of tests and I was frightened, but Mum and I had a lot of support from the Nurses and Doctors. Mum was allowed to stay in a bed next to me, because we came from Devon. During my stay there I had a P.H. Study and an Endoscopy, so my movement was quite restricted, but the ward's play leader kept me busy. The playroom was very good, and had lots of games and videos. It also had a Nintendo with lots of video games to play on it. During my stay on Dickens I did make some friends which made my stay easier. When I was told I had IBD I didn't understand what it meant. It was explained to me by pictures, by a Staff Nurse called Crispen. I now understand all about my disease. My Doctor, Dr Hill put me on some drugs to control my IBD. I still have IBD, and have ruff patches, and have to take lots of medicine to keep me healthy. I get tired and cold very easily, but as long as I am careful, I can keep fit and healthy.

Stephi Reynolds, age 13

Dear William.
My thoughts on GOSH.   Mark Evans.

I first went to GOSH when I was 11 months old in January 1988 when it was still the Old Hospital and I stayed in ward 1B. The nurses in charge then were Lindy & Kim. I was rushed in to GOSH by ambulance suffering with Hydrocephalus, and I had my First operation then. On that first stay I was in hospital for a week.
I returned for another operation 4 years later and have had many operations since, I am now 14 years old.
    The old ward was very cramped but the nurses were fantastic. When the new part of the hospital was opened and the patients were transferred to the new Parrot Ward it was amazing the amount of room and facilities compared to the old ward Was unbelievable.
    I have known many nurses and have had my stays in hospital made much more Enjoyable because of them and their happy faces. Some of them are: Lindy, Kim, Harry, Melissa, Stephanie, Fiona, Sally, Charlotte and Play Specialists Sarah & Jo. I have met a few famous people who have come and visited which was very nice.
    The school and playrooms are very friendly and has many things to play and Do, the best thing about them is that you are out of bed and off the ward for a while.
    I made some friends over the years who we still keep in touch with.
Many thanks to people like William who give up their time to visit sick children like me.
    Mark Evans.

Mark Evans, age 14

208

Dec 01/01

My name is Scott Fitzmaurice and I live in Essex. I am 14yrs old and I have been coming to Great Ormond Street Hospital since I was 1yr old. I have problems with my right leg. It is a lot shorter than my left leg. I also my ACL and PCL ligaments are missing in my knee.
I have had six operations so far and expect to have quite a few more. My first Consultant was Mr Fixen but he retired so Mr Monsell and his team now look after me. My last operation was just a few weeks ago, I was on the ward for 8 days because I had an abscess grow on a couple of my old pin sights. I always stay on Clarence Ward, the nurses are always happy. I had my first operation when I was 8yrs old to lengthen my right leg. Some of nurses that looked after me then back in 1995 are still working on the ward now.
My Consultant Mr Monsell supports Tottenham and I support Sheffield Wednesday so we always wined each other up about it.

Scott Fitzmaurice, age 14

Great Ormond Street **NHS**
Hospital for Children
NHS Trust

Great Ormond Street
London WC1N 3JH

Tel: 020 7405 9200

I am on Badger ward. I am 14 years old. I come to GOSH every month for IV x antibiotics. I have a the lot. of freinds up here. The nurses are nice. I like comedy. The hospital food is un-appetising. William is a ~~nice~~ very nice man.

Dominic King

IV   intravenous

In Partnership with the Institute of Child Health, UCL
Patron: Her Majesty The Queen
Chairman: Sir Cyril Chantler MA MD FRCP FRCPCH FMedSci

Dominic King, age 14

10-8-02

102 wind mill Rd
Hemel Hempstead
Hart. Hp2 4Bw

Bear william
I read your diary. I enjoyed
It very much. my Dad thinks It is very
good. It reminded my of some of my
friends.
Since my Lung and heart tiansplant
I have been getting on well

Lot's of Love
AJay macleilan
x x x

AJay McClellan, age 14

Siobhán Morris age 14 next Saturday 12th January

Every 2-3 months I spend 2 weeks in Great Ormond Street Hospital to have intrevenous antibiotics, intensive physio here (who make me work) and try to avoid the clowns and the school teachers. I have Cystic fibrosis so I'm quite high maintenance - trying to prevent chest infections. On my birthday (for which I'm unfortunatly admitted) I plan to do lunch with my play specialists Lizzie and Amy. Being in this hospital is unlike being in any other hospital, the walls on my ward are lined with badgers, people are very freindly and there isn't a smell of disenfectant or soup anywhere.

Siobhán Morris, age 14

My name is Nicholas Petrie. In 1997 I was diagnosed with Non Hodgkin's t-cell lymphoma. My treatment was spread over two long years and it was shared between GOSH and The Royal Free Hospital. They treated me with chemotherapy, a mixture of powerful drugs. I spent more time at the Royal Free than at GOSH. but being ill was 'better' at GOSH rather than the Royal Free because I could roam around the ward and make friends and play snooker and chat with friends because every one at GOSH on Lion ward was being treated for similar illnesses. But at the Royal Free there was the general side as well where there were people who had broken legs and the flu and I could catch flu and die because the drugs I was having made me weak.

I met William when I was in hospital for a routine part of my treatment, I used to have banners on my door saying who I was, and William came in and introduced him self. We became goods friends both being Chelsea supporters and he brought me back a programme from the 1997 F.A. cup final and a Chelsea watch. We were also featured in an article William wrote for The Roundabout, the Gosh magazine.

Whilst in GOSH I started to collect badges and pencils and William gave me many badges and pencils for my collection. One badge is very, very special as it is the actual badge that he wore to Princess Diana's funeral, William was asked to attend as a representative of GOSH.

During my treatment there were ups and downs. It was very important for me to be able to look on the bright side of life and to enjoy my self even whilst I was in hospital but especially when I was at home with my friends. It was always nice to see a different face whilst I was in hospital instead of just the nurses and my Mum and my Dad. William always brought a smile to my face.

During my second year of treatment I did not spend as much time as an in-patient at GOSH, but attended Elephant ward , we would usually see William as he worked on the front desk at that time I remember he would always give me some pocket money to spend.

I would also like to say thank you to my Mum Dad all the Nurses and Doctors and both GOSH and the Royal Free.

Nicholas Petrie, age 14

My Thoughts On Great Ormond Street
Hospital

Hello, my name is Emma kate Upson age 14. I've been coming

to GOSH since I was about 4 years old (about 10 years). In 1996, the

doctors discovered I had Perthes disease in my hips. I had to have 3

operations; the first to test what was wrong; the second to replace the hip

and to place a pin and plate in it; and the third to remove the pin and plate.

After I had had my second operation and had my plaster off for a week I fell over

in the sitting room on my crutches and broke my thema (just above the knee) and

was in plaster for another twelve weeks. Just after I had had my second

operation my little brother Michael was born too.

I was in Clarence ward for all 3 operations and my nurse happened

to be a man called Terry, he was very funny and made me laugh.

William also came to visit me on his rounds, this made me very

happy as William is a very nice man indeed and helped me get

through my operations.

In 1998, I was also on ITN News at 1, demonstrating the new

morphine pain relief button. Mum was feeding Michael and

popped her head around the curtain because she thought

they'd finished filming, but they hadn't. My teddy-Old Bear

was lying next to me during filming too. He is nearly 200 years

Emma Upson, age 14

I was also on radio GOSH and said a few words on it to cheer people up who could not go up there for various reasons and I played some music too. I was lucky enough to be able to go to the GOSH School too. On one of the days we had a static electricity science lesson and I tested out a experiment; they stuck two balloons to the side of my head at the end and I went away for lunch. They stayed on for about an hour and then fell off; me, my mum and my dad stuck them back on just before the afternoon session and tricked the teacher and other pupils. On the second day an actor from CATS came to visit and showed us her hand-made wig.

Another thing they had was a scout, guide and brownie club. This was pretty much the same as anywhere else but it was still good fun. I went along and joined in. They also have playrooms for little children to keep them happy.

At GOSH they also have a physio therapy pool which is good fun and great exercise and they have a gym to exercise in too. All the physiotherapists there, I thought were lovely too.

My thoughts on gosh are that nobody wants to be in hospital, but if you have to GOSH is the place to be. I doubt you could find a better hospital than GOSH in the world.

by Emma Kate Upson. 17/12/01.

Emma Upson

Dialysis Unit,
Great Ormond Street

25th July 2002

My name is Michael Anderton and I am 15 years old.
I attend Great. Ormond. Street Hospital because
I have to have Haemodialysis as I dont
have any working kidneys. I come to Gosh
3 days a week to have dialysis. In the dialysis
Unit everyone is really friendly, both fellow patients
and staff. Hopefully one day, I will get a kidney
transplant and will no longer have to attend
Great Ormond Street Hospital.

Michael Anderton, 15

Michael Anderton, age 15

Dear William,

I was delighted to hear that your diary has sold so well. I have written a short article, which I hope you can use for the extra pages, which is enclosed. Have a wonderful Christmas and New Year, It's lovely that you have chosen to change your plans so that you can go to GOSH and help cheer up those who aren't lucky enough to be at home.

Best wishes

Sarah /x

Sarah Carvosso, age 15

Living with someone elses heart is a rather hard concept to grasp but one I had to accept after undergoing a heart transplant at Great ormond street in September 2001 due to the unexpected contraction of Cardio Myopathy. Unlike most teenagers I now face a life of check-ups, pills and pharmacutical bills which was certainly a daunting prospect for me, as a person who has hardly ever been ill in my life before. However, thanks to the doctors and nurses at GOSH I have now come to terms with the fact that this is what my life entails but at the same time realised that they can be factors which are very much in the background of a normal life.

I was in GOSH for a very long and hard 3 months and aswell as my fantastic family and friends it was the nurses who got me through. Weather it was their gossip, jokes, holiday stories or guy chat they always managed to cheer me up and became like friends.

I met some of the bravest children too, who have had the most horrific childhoods due to their illnesses and I now appreciate how lucky was to have had such a healthy life up until now. They have made the most of life despite their troubles and have not let illness beat their bubbly charaters.

Considdering when I came round from my 8 hour opperation I couldn't walk, talk or eat without the aid of a tube, I have made remarkable progress. I am now at home and beginning to get back to school and go out and about with friends like I used to.

Although I would never have asked for this to happen it enabled me to meet lots of great people and the experience taught me to live life to the full as you never know what's around the next corner' by Sarah Carvosso, 15

Sarah Carvosso

DARREN OSGOOD.

Dear William.

I have been going to G.O.S for 11 years, I have been into G.O.S many times to have test done to find out what Condition I have. After many years I found out the name of my condition. I have myotonic Dystrophy. Mytonic Dystrophy is muscle weakness and wasting due to the muscle weakness. I get very tierd and can only do parttime at school, I have to rest every day at school and at home. My body lets me down a lot and every 4 to 5 weeks my body Just will not go on and I have to rest for 2 weeks and their nothing I can do Just rest. I have dietary Problem, I cannot have Dairy, wheat, Eggs, Soya. I have a Gastroenteri bottom in my tummy which I have to vent from 3 times a day and I have a night feed. Last time I was in G.O.S was in July 2001 for a bad cough I had. At G.O.S I see DR Lindley Gastroenterology clinic DR C. Devile Neurology clinic. and DR M Bryon who is with the respiratory team. DR Lindley I have known for many years he has helped me a lot and he makes me laugh. I have been to the hospital school and I liked it very much, I like the food they do for my diet. The Nurse's are very nice and so are the doctors. G.O.S does not smell like a hospital. Next time I go to G.O.S is Febuary 4th, I go to G.O.S a lot. Their is allways a nice friendley face to wellcome you and William you play a lot in that.

Sincerley Darren OSGOOD

Darren Osgood, age 15

Great Ormond Street
Hospital for Children
NHS Trust

Great Ormond Street
London WC1N 3JH

Tel: 020 7405 9200

My name is nathan and i am 16 yrs old. GOSH is a very nice hospital I am on Badger ward The nurses are great, I Like all the nurses because they are treat me with care. The hospital food is ok, i like it. William is a very nice man he has gave lots of things So if there was an award for the kindest man i think He would win it. Great ormond street hospital is a Good Hospital. Some of the Doctors are nice except a few with names I can't recall. I have a illness called cystic Fibrosos and i come into hospital every 3months for 2weeks for IV antibitics I have lots of friends My two best friends are on Badger Ward are Dominic King lothan and Abdul Aslam.
Blizzard-welch.
Physio is Good when you can go to the gym or go swimming
I like esta

In Partnership with the Institute of Child Health, UCL
Patron: Her Majesty The Queen
Chairman: Sir Cyril Chantler MA MD FRCP FRCPCH FMedSci

Nathan Blizzard-Welch, age 16

Thoughts on Great Ormond Street

In search of help is why I came
To get me fixed, to feel no more pain
I wonder why, these people care
I wonder why, these people are there
Fat or thin, black or white
These people devote their life to make us right
They're there every second of every day
So take a moment to hear what I have to say
I say thank you to every doctor and every nurse
And I'd like to say my love and time has been put into every
verse.

Thank you
Marc Dickson

Marc Dickson, age 16

27th December 2001

Dear William

I am sorry that I never wrote back straight away, but I have enclosed a poem about Great Ormond Street, I am sixteen now and will be visiting the hospital during the next few weeks, possibly for the last time as I am now getting too old to attend a children's hospital.

I will never forget the care and attention that the doctors and nurses give to each and every child, they strive to make our stays in the hospital as pleasant as possible and make us feel as special as they can.

I have a kidney disease that will never go away, but the doctors have done their best for me to make me understand what is wrong and how to live my life the best I can without making things worse for myself.

I have written many poems like the one which I have enclosed for you, some are about my life and others are about the things that I love, I do hope that you can publish my poem in your new book, as I would love to see one of my poems with my name in print.

William, do take care, hope to hear from you soon.

Marc.

Marc Dickson

My name is Sophia El-kaddah I have Cerebral Palsy Quadraplegia. I have been receiving treatment at Great Ormond Street Hospital since I was 2yrs old. Cerebral Palsy Quadraplegia means that I was starved of oxygen at birth, and due to this I received some brain damage which resulted in me having Cerebral palsy.

I initially went to Great Ormond Street to have my hips put back into their sockets and later I began receiving treatment for my back. I endure alot of pain on a daily basis because of my spine.

I first met William during a two month stay on Clarence ward where he would come and visit sick children. When William used to come to the ward he always put a smile on my face even when I was in unbearable pain. I also made some friends during that 2mths among them were the nurses Mel, Terry and Keith. I still keep in touch with Mel even though she has left the ward and I write regularly to William.

Sophia El-Kaddah, age 16

223

My name is Mark Hawkins I have been affiliated with
G.O.S.H My whole life, since I was diagnosed with cystic
fibrosis in fact.

I used to attend my local hospital (barnet general) untill my
condition grew more serious and great ormond street hospital
was the best place to go to for my IVs. i think i was 6~7 year
old.

Being a patient at G.O.S has changed my life I used to
be quite a thin small person and the doctors and nurses
here have helped me develop more.

Sometimes the doctors and nurses can ~~be a bit much about~~
~~certain things that they believe are good for us, that in fact~~
~~are not~~ not understand that some forms of medication
help in body but not in spirit.

Even though I'd like to I will not mention my favaroute
nurses cos' that wouldn't be fair, but I think nearly every
nurse here on badger ~~ward~~ ward (formerly Alexandre ward)
and all over the hospital are really caring and pleasent people,
They always try to make life better for you even if it
doesn't look like it (i.e. Feed chart).

Great ormond street hospital isn't just a place to get
medication it's a place where you can come on a little
holiday from home. I think most kids bring in their
favaroute toys, games, music or other fun things they use.
Compared to an adult hospital G.O.S.H is such a place
of more happiness.

I have met alot of other Teenagers with the same
condition i have thanks to G.O.S and each time
i come in for a two week IV course there is usually
another CF (cystic fibrosis) patient my age in.
When i met these guys ~~━━━━━━~~ I was a bit nervous
but then i realised these guys go through the same
bad things and good that i go through.
Each time i come in it's like a reunion of ~~old friends~~
friends and we can play on games or just chat
anytime.
Me and ~~✱~~ Abdul and Dominic and Johnathon
used to have chess tournaments.

Mark Hawkins, age 16

I remember one time when Me an Abdul got in trouble with the nurses for writing on papers and sticking them to the window that seperated our two rooms so when the other looked in he would see a sign reading something like "~~that something~~ ~~is that~~) "Stop reading this and get back to work". The reason we got in trouble is because we went overboard and put signs all over the ward.

The reason i think i remember times like this is because it's times like these and times like when me and Jay mcleanon had a few wheel chair races that you can forget why you're in hospital and Just have fun.

William Gates the man who wrote this book is a remarkable man, he is the type of Person who gives and gives and doesn't think of any reward. In todays day and age a person like William is more race than anything you can imagine. From what i have seen William is a man who is kind no matter what.

Great Ormond Street Hospital is a hospital but it's so welcoming and comfortable that it's hard to leave.

~~Mark~~

Mark Anthony Hawkins, 16,

Mark Hawkins

Thoughts
on GOSH

I've Been Coming 2 Gosh
Since I woc 2 months old.
The hospital hasn't changed
that much other than new
wards. have been added* I have
met a docter to be called
emily who came round the
ward in order to get to
know people before she becomes
a docter. I have brittle bones
which means my bones break
quite easily and so I have
been to many wards and
have met a lot of people
but each ward I have been
to all the staff have been
helpful and willing to help me Great ormond
street is great.   Marc Lambert 16 yrs old.

Marc Lambert, age 16

226

8/1/02

Dear William Gates

Hello how are you I hope you
are fine and Thankyou for the letter
you sent me you are my best friend
william and I have to go to school on
the 8th January and I am going to Pizza
Hut on The 10th January with my friends
because it is my Kidneys birthday it
is going to be 3 years old on 10th January
and I really want to buy a Soft toy
dog I am Saving my Poctet money
it is for £14.99 I really would like
that for my Kidneys birthday because
it is very Soft I love it and it
is in mother care and they said
adopt a Puppy dog from mother care and
I have not bean Well because having bead Pan
head pain
            Thankyou

            Love
            from

            Shabnam
            Malik

Shabnam Malik, age 16

I found out I had chronic renal failure when I was 8 years old.
I started dialysis in 1995 which my mum done for me.Then I had my first
kidney transplant in 1996 I caught glandular fever and lost the kidney I
was in hospital for 4 months.My secound transplant was in 1998 I
caught the cmv virus.i struggled to keep my kidney for 2 months.
Im 16 now and living a normal live expect the fact I have to drink 2 litres
a day,take loads of tablets and give myself an injection once a week.but
that is nothing in comparision to what some of the other ill children
have to go through.Looking back it was a very emotional time for me
and I wont lie when I say that it was a very painful time aswell but it
saved my life which I,m very grateful for because I love my family so
much I cant bear to leave them.I don't have the words to thank the
nurses and doctors who have helped me emotionally and physically i
will be eternally grateful.There are some days when I feel sorry for
myself but in some ways I,m glad I have an illness [yes I know it sounds
weird]but it has taught me a lot of knowledge over the past few years
about myself,people and how powerful the human spirit can be.I guess
sometimes I feel like I have been given a gift and I,m meant to use my
gift to help other people.I figure lifes a gift and I don't intend on
wasting it.

Michelle nichols
Age.16 years

Michelle Nichols, age 16

21st January, Monday

Dear William;

Sorry it has taken me so long to write to you, please forgive me. I have been unbeleivably busy. As I said when I saw you last Tuesday, exams and the preperatition has taken up most of my time. Now that I'm back at school the time is flying, as I have an unbelievable amount of work to do. I am working very hard as my exam results can only help me in life. My teachers have said that I am on target and with some extra hard work should do quite well. I haven't long left as I leave at the middle of may time and go back in June for my exams!

I will hopefully be getting a small part time job. It is only saturdays, but some thing to start me off, I shall hopefully be working as a sales assistant, selling school uniforms to small children. It would be the ideal job for me. The shop hasn't opened yet, it is the National School wear Centre, or something similar, I have already spoken to the manager and he said he shall send me an application form. That was friday. If was not arrived by tomorrows mail I ~~thing~~ think I may phone up again. I shall try very hard and I am eager to start.

I am reading the book you sent me at the moment, I am yet to finish it. I had no idea you were such an accomplished author. I have always wanted to write, I must have started at least a hundred stories/novels, but

James Warman, age 16

have never finished any. I am filled with excitement of the prospect of my job. I shall write you any news I get on that subject. My aunt recently had a baby. So many of my mother's friends are expecting or have recently giving birth. It is such a privelege to see a new born life.

If I get this job, then I shall modify my aviary greatly and get some new birds. One of them still has your name on it.

I was not sure on what you wanted me to write, I'm afraid I lost the guide line, but I shall hopefully have not left any thing out.

I first had my 'illness' when i was 9 years old. unfortunately, although my local hospital was very good they did not know what was wrong with me, so there, was not much they could do about it.

It was late December, early January an my situation was bad. One of the nurses suggested I went to great Ormond Street, Hospital for Sick Children. I remember very little of when I was transferred as I drifted in and out of conciousness. The doctors at GOSH, were able to diagnose me straight away with Stevens Johnsons Syndrome (SJS). Doctor Atherton and his team were very good. They put me on a dosage of steroids and the swelling in the face and lips went down almost immeadiatley. After a few days I was put on to slice words They are very good their. My nurse on the first night was Fiona. She was wonderful and very kind, but strict, but that only helped my recovery.

James Warman

The teachers got me working almost right away, which was good. The play specialist Louisa, got me motivated and playing games, which was great, because with out her I would have just stayed in bed feeling sorry for myself.

One time, my mum, was talking in reception, to a gentle man named William. She mentioned that I wouldn't have any visitors that evening and so he came to visit me. I was so pleased, and made a very good friend in William who came to see me often, he found out that Wine Gums are my favourites and he kindly brought me some whenever I was leaving. Over the years to many times I have been in GOSH, William never once missed seeing me.

Great Ormond Street Hospital, the people in it helped me so much, and i have been in the clear for nearly 2 years. I made some very good friends their and shall never forget their kindness, most of all my parents love and support.

I hope that is ok william and every thing you need is their.

I shall write you soon,
Take care of yourself.
See you soon

James Warman.

James Warman

Dg. Dialsis Unit

Dear Will

Hi my name is Fred Ayisi and I been coming to
GOSH for 15 year now I am 17 year ~~of age~~ old. I
like Gosh because it has loads of activies like
the Den and computer night at ~~school~~.

~~Af~~ There are loads of friendly people in gosh
I would name them out it will ~~~~ take two
pages
This was a great idea to do a ~~~~ book on children

Thanks Will.

Fred Ayisi (17)

Fred Ayisi, age 17

232

16.7.02

Dear William,

I have been coming to GOSH since I was three years old, I have osteogenesis imperfecta (Type III) which means my bones are weak. At the moment I'm in Dickens ward, having treatment to increase my bone density.

I find GOSH a very friendly environment. The nurses, doctors etc are excellent in what they do. The nurses are helpful and kind, the doctors are understanding and have answered my questions fully. The teachers at the hospital school, are helpful and don't make it boring (which means I can not escape my schoolwork!). The other staff members are friendly too. The only thing I don't like is the food! GOSH has helped me a lot and I think its one of the Hospital's I've been to.

Over the years I have made many friends. When I had my first infusion I met Mark and his mum. Mark has the same condition as me. Mark is funny and we get along great.

Few months ago I met William who is lovely. He was telling me that he was writing a diary. When I read it, I couldn't put it down. Its mostly about children coming to GOSH to have operations etc.

Take care.

Lots of Love

Meesha Patel 17yrs old.

- x -

GOSH IS GREAT

Meesha Patel, age 17

I am Byron Rawlings, now 17 years old. When I was 15 I was a normal outgoing teenager when in the summer of 99 I noticed my stomach had got very large and that I was getting tired quickly. I kept this quiet for a while but one day my mum noticed this and insisted that I go down to the doctors. The doctor told me that I had fluid inside my stomach and I was immediately placed in the Norfolk and Norwich hospital. I was in there for about a week and on medicine to make me go to the toilet lots. After a week Dr Julian Eason told me that I was in Heart Failure. Then after a few tests and a day visit to GOSH I was assigned to go there for surgery. When I got to GOSH I thought that the odds on my operation were 99% fine. My illness was confirmed as Calcification of the periocardium which means that the sack around the heart had gone hard. I didn't want to know what the operation was about or the odds so I didn't listen but found out afterwards that the odds had gone from 99% to 60% survival. I was in GOSH for about 10 days and all the staff were brilliant. I do remember a nice nurse called Niere who I think was a trainee. I have now got the all clear and never have to visit a hospital for a check up again. GOSH is a wonderfull place and everyone there does a great job especially William Gates!

Byron Rawlings, age 17

234

19.12.200

My Time in Great Ormond Street Hospital!

My name is Barry Stapleton and I was amitted to G.O.S.H in December 1996. I was twelve years old, I had A.L.L Leukaemia. I was referred from Barnet General Hospital where I stayed for five weeks, they could not find out what was the matter with me.

Having leukaemia was very hard and difficult and being in G.O.S.H for so long was emotionally draining, but it had to be done and I had to get through it. My treatment for my illness was chemotherapy inserted in a Hickman line and a course of Lumberpuntures inserted in to my spine. I was in G.O.S.H for one year, I am fully recovered now and I am just taking each day as it comes. My consultant at the time of my illness was Dr. Michalski. It wasn't pleasant being in hospital but G.O.S.H made it a lot easier to cope with, e.g. the gym, my own room and my own TV and video & bathroom.

I made some close friends in hospital but many of the children in the hospital were babies & toddlers. We were all very ill. One day a voluntary worker called William Gates came to see me and over the course of the year we became good friends, I looked forward to William visiting me, he played an important part in my stay in hospital. We see each other quite regularly at important occasions such as my confirmation, birthdays, football matches and hope to remain friends for a long, long time to come.

I am now seventeen years old. My next appointment is in June 2002 and if that goes well I will be five years away from treatment and the hospital have assured me that if every thing is ok, I am in the clear.

Never give up there's always hope!

Barry Stapleton
Barry stapleton

1

Barry Stapleton, age 17

Index

A

237

B

Baker, Craig	Patient, Elephant Day Care, 39
Baker, Marjorie	Wife of Cyril, 124,142
Baker, Cyril	Friend, 142
Bannach, Ellen	Librarian, Jena University, Germany, 110, 114, 158
Barrar, Saskia	Outpatient 130
Bastin, John	Father of Andrew, 39
Bastin, Helen	Wife of John, 39
Bastin, Hannah	Daughter of John & Helen, 39
Bastin, Andrew	Outpatient, Brother of Hannah, 39
Baxter, Chelsea	Patient, Alexandra Ward, 100, 134, 135, 137
Baxter, Mary	Mother of Chelsea, 135
Beck, Lily	Patient, Fox Ward, 115, 116
Bedane, Albert	Channel Island WW2 hero, 84
Bennett, Ted	Royal Mid-Surrey Golf Club, 113, 124, 135
Bennett, Glen	Wife of Ted, 113, 124, 135
Bibby, Sandy	Friend, 64
Bibby, Constance	Wife of Sandy, 64
Black, Stephanie	Business Manager, Lloyds Bank, 134
Black, Stanley	Dance Band leader, 41
Blake, Naomi	Sculptor, 67
Blair, Tony	Prime Minister, 16, 101
Blanks, Don	Brother of Sylvia Gates, 122
Blanks, Doreen	Twin sister of Don, 122
Blizzard-Welch, Nathan	Patient, Alexandra Ward, 43, 45, 47
Boag, Adam	Outpatient,17
Bonhoeffer, Dietrich	German Lutherian, executed by Nazis, 50, 118
Booth, Jack	Patient, Victoria Ward, 24
Borham, Alex	Patient, Churchill Ward, 80
Boys, Rex	Neighbour, 94, 95
Boys, Dickerle	Wife of Rex, 94, 95
Bradbury,Malcolm	Writer, 142
Bradley	Patient with special needs, 91
Brady, Laura	Patient, 91
Brainwood, Peter	President, Grays Thurroch Rotary Club, 18
Brian	Racing promoter, 156
Brown, Patrick	Patient, Annie Zunz Ward, 113
Buck, Harry	Patient, Lion Ward, 148
Burch, Emily	Patient, Lion Ward, 59
Bush, George	President, United States of America, 130
Butler, Lord	Former Home Secretary, 142

C

Caly	Patient, Victoria Ward, 100
Candarli, Osman	Patient, Parrot Ward, 71
Caplin, Celia	Neighbour, 93
Caplin, Irving	Son of Celia, 93
Caplin, Rene	Sister of Celia, 93
Carr, Jake	Patient, Lion Ward, 125
Cartright, Freddie	Elephant Day Care, 77
Cavalli, Ben	Patient, Alexandra Ward, 17, 19, 20, 21, 23, 24, 25, 32, 36, 38, 42, 52, 74, 86, 94, 95, 96, 97, 98, 101, 102, 103, 112, 114, 116, 121, 126, 136
Cecil, Andrew	Patient, Clarence Ward, 79, 84, 99
Chambers, John James	President, Liverpool Beatles Appreciation Society, 29
Chang, Michael	Patient, Hedgehog Ward, 52
Chantelle	Patient, Clarence Ward, 126
Charlie	Patient, Tiger Ward, 23
Charlesworth, Marian	Friend, 137
Chessinton World of Adventures	14. See Grove International, 17
Chick, Albert	Friend, 95, 98, 102
Chick, Doll	Wife of Alby, 95, 98, 102
Chick, Steve	Son of Alby, 95, 98
Chick, James	Son of Steve & Sally, 95
Chick, Sarah	Sister of James, 95
Chung, Kai	Father of Anita Weinel, 24
Chung, Irene	Wife of Kai, 24
Church, Steven	Outpatient, 42, 51, 52, 75, 77
Clark, Alan	MP & writer,156
Clark, Nigel	Chairman, Fundraising, 154
Cliffe, Ros	Director, Fundraising, 116
Cloe	School friend of Heather Munro, 157
Cochrane, Ian	Writer, 142
Codrai, Janet	Daughter of Alby & Doll Chick, 95
Cole, Nicholas	Patient, Clarence Ward, 82, 91, 97, 99, 117, 148
Cole, Samantha	Mother of Nicholas, 82, 97, 99, 117, 148
Collins, James	Marks & Spencer, Pantheon, 145
Collins, Susan	Daughter of Nettie Rolnick, 20, 68
Collins, Michael	Husband of Sue, 92
Collins, Derek	Former executive, Lloyds Bank, 31,73, 92, 134
Collins, Pamela	Wife of Derek, 31, 73
Collins, Matthew	Uncle of Birmingham teenagers killed in fire, 44

Doubleday, Isobel	Wife of John, 11, 26, 27, 31, 34, 50, 69, 82, 92, 116, 134, 146
Doubleday, Robert	Son of John & Isobel, 11, 27, 28, 31, 34, 50, 51, 52, 69, 82, 92, 157
Doubleday, Edwin	Brother of Robert, 11, 26, 27, 28, 31, 32, 33, 34, 38, 42, 45, 50, 52, 64, 69, 76, 77, 82, 92, 116, 146, 157
Doubleday, James	Brother of Robert & Edwin, 11, 26, 27, 34, 50, 51, 82, 157
Doubleday, Andrew	Brother of John, 31
Doubleday, George	Son of Andrew, 31
Doubleday, William	Brother of George, 31
Doubleday, Tom	Brother of George & William, 31
Doyle-Davidson, Richard	Former Managing Director, Wentworth Golf Club, 124
Doyle-Davidson, Barbara	Wife of Richard, 31, 124
Doyle, Wendy	Social Worker, 20, 22, 23, 24, 36
Dullah, Nina	Staff Nurse, David Waterson Ward, 19, 34, 86
Duncan, Nishka	Patient, Clarence Ward, 53, 55
Dunn, James	Patient, Alice Ward, 39
Dunne, Liam	Patient, PICU, 59
Dum Family	Killed by Nazis WW2, 67
Durie, Ian, The Rev.	Former Brigadier. Uncle of Edwin Doubleday, 77
Durie, Sarianne	Sister of Isobel Doubleday, 77

E

Easter, Tim	Organist, former patient, 154
Edwards, Adam	Patient, Victoria Ward, 49
Edwards, Christopher	Friend,155
Edwards, Betty	Wife of Chris, 34
El Kaddah, Sophia	Patient, Clarence Ward, 48, 49, 100, 107, 109, 120, 121, 123
Ellis, Christopher	Patient, Victoria Ward, 79, 102
Eton, Sotiris	Patient, Fox Ward, 51, 53, 54, 55, 57, 59, 72, 75, 95, 98
Evans, Mark	Patient, Parrot Ward, 111
Everett, Marie	Daughter of Rosie Watts, 41, 55, 56, 57, 66, 129
Everett, Brian	Husband of Marie, 57
Everett, Thomas	Patient, Alexandra Ward, 126, 128
Evers, Sarah	Patient, David Waterson Ward,123

F

G

Gauston, Matthew	Patient, Clarence Ward,15
Gavin, Tom	Grandson of Frances Delaney, 89
Geffen, Edward	Patient, Parrot Ward, 113, 119, 121
Geffen, Camilla	Mother of Edward, 113, 119
Geffen, Robin	Father of Edward, 119
Geistfeld, Loren	Professor, University of Ohio, U.S.A., 83, 107
Geistfeld, Carol	Wife of Loren, 83
Georgeou, Micheal	Dental Surgeon, R.D. McKennell, 68, 133
Georgina	Mother's lodger in Hampton Wick, 41
Gibson, Timothy	Patient, David Waterson Ward, 72, 75, 77
Gielgud, Sir John	Actor, 70
Gilbert, Zak	Patient, Fox Ward, 13, 70, 72, 75, 90, 100, 101, 102, 108
Gilbert, Martin	Father of Zak, 90, 100, 101
Gilbert, Lorraine	Wife of Martin, 100
Gilbert, Ben	School friend of Sean Robinson, 108
Gladden, Vanessa	Patient, Robin Ward, 19, 80, 86
Gladden, Sue	Mother of Vanessa, 80
Gleek, Norman	Friend of Nettie Rolnick, 99
Goader, Edward	Patient, Clarence Ward, 123
Goldner, Karima	Patient, PICU, 134, 135
Goldner, Mafedha	Mother of Karima,134
Goldner, Khalid	Brother of Karima, 134, 135
Goodwin, Aubrey	Past Captain, Royal Mid-Surrey Golf Club, 58
Goodwin, Dianna,	Wife of Aubrey, 58
Goodwin, Anthony	Son of Aubrey & Dianna, 58
Goodwin, Pat	Wife of Anthony, 58
GOSH	Great Ormond Street Hospital
Gore, Al	Vice-President, United States of America, 130
Green, Laurence	Nephew of Celia Caplin, 93
Green, Richard	Godfather of Edward Geffen, 119
Greenman, Leon	Survivor of Auschwitz, 12, 93, 153
Greenman, Barney	Son of Leon. Murdered in Auschwitz, 93
Gregorowski, Anna	Sister, Alice Ward, 132, 133, 140, 141
Gregory & Radice	Literary Agent, 12, 13, 14, 16
Gregov, Kevin	Patient, Tiger Ward, 47
Grosher, Lydia	Patient, Fox Ward, 139
Gross, Dr	Nazi Medical Professor who experimented on, and killed, handicapped children, 43, 44
Grostate, Millie	Reception, Front Desk, 18, 40, 94, 126
Grove, Mr	Chairman, Grove International, 17
Groves, Dale	Patient, Parrot Ward, 47
Grosvenor, Stephen	Patient, Louis Ward, 39, 46, 52
Grosvenor, Julie	Mother of Stephen, 46

H

Jones, Keith	Husband of Kay, 101
Jones, Michelle	Patient, Lion Ward, 59, 60, 61, 63, 64, 70
Jones, Chris	Father of Michelle, 64
Jones, Sarah	Wife of Chris, 60, 70
Jones, Stephanie	Sister of Michelle, 59, 64
Jones, Gemma	Daughter of Jane Weinel, 62, 82,108, 117, 157
Jones, Hayden,	Son of Gemma, 105, 108, 117, 157
Jones, Charmaine	Marks & Spencer, Pantheon, 145
Jordan, William	Patient, Helena Ward, 46, 47, 49, 101, 102, 103
Jordan, Tracey	Mother of William, 101, 102
Judith	Consultant, 15

K

Kaker, Yasmin	Marks & Spencer, Pantheon, 145, 149
Karou	Japanese Student, 106
Kate	Staff Nurse, Robin Ward, 34
Kearns, Joan	Manager, Fundraising, 58, 60
Keegan, Dr	Consultant, Moorfields Eye Hospital, 138
Kei	Japanese Student, 106
Keogh, Adam	Outpatient, 129
Kerrie	Staff Nurse, Robin Ward, 35
Kev	Carer, Barnardo's, 107
Khan, Aleena	Patient, Parrot Ward, 123, 126
Khartoon, Ayisha	Patient, Dialysis, 45
Khatum, Halima	Patient, Clarence Ward, 45
Khwaja, Haroon	Ahmadujya Youth Association, 58
Kibblewhite, Ashley	Friend, 127
Kibblewhite, Anya	Wife of Ashley, 127
King, Dave	Fire Officer, 140
King, Dominic	Patient, Alexandra Ward, 39, 43, 45, 154
King, Diana	Mother of Dominic, 154
Koker, Mehmet	Patient, Dialysis and Victoria Ward, 14, 53, 75, 79, 95
Koprivica, Zoran	Manager, Food, Marks & Spencer, Pantheon, 145
Kuladie, Nichesh	Patient, Victoria Ward, 111

L

La	Reception, Front Desk, 137
Lambert, Marc	Patient, Clarence Ward, 82, 84
Larson, Fitz	Husband of Clare, 94
Larson, Clare	Sister of Richard Leslie, 94

246

N

Nash, Matthew	Patient, Lion Ward, 57
Neame, Alan	Friend, Writer, 116, 132, 137, 138, 156
Newland, Michael, Dr.	General Practitioner, 92, 94, 124
Ngala, Lydia	Patient, Robin Ward, 135
Nguyen, Michael	Patient, Parrot Ward, 61, 65
Nguyen, Esther	Mother of Michael, 61, 65
Nguyen, Tian	Marks & Spencer, Pantheon,145
Nia	Patient, Parrot Ward, 59
Nichols, Michelle	Patient, Victoria Ward, 153
Nicholson, Sheila	Friend, 99
Nielson, Dennis	Serial killer, 21
Nietzsche, Friedrich	German philosopher & poet, 62, 63
Nott, Mr	Consultant, Westminister & Chelsea Hospital, 82
Nugent, Kevin,	Patient, Elephant Day Care, 113
Nussbraum, Tzvl,	Jewish boy arrested by Nazis, Warsaw, WW2, 67

O

O'Connor, Charlotte	Patient, Fox Ward, 59
O'Connor, Des	Des O'Connor Show, ITV, 46, 47, 48, 49, 58, 59
O'Gorman, Elizabete	Sports Centre, Dolphin Square, 127
O'Grady, Kathy	Marks & Spencer, Pantheon, 46, 92, 145, 157
Ogden, Richard	Patient, Alexandra Ward, 39
Olivier	French Teacher killed in car accident, 49
Open, Marc	Stepfather of Ben Cavalli, 74
Owens, Pauric	Outpatient, 121
Oxland, Carol	Mother of Laura Brady, 91

P

Page, Ronnie	Manager, Sports Centre, Dolphin Square, 81, 101, 121, 128, 146, 155
Page, Dianne,	Wife of Ronnie, 101, 121
Page, Katie	Daughter of Ronnie & Dianne, 101, 121
Page, William	Brother of Katie, 101, 121
Paine, David	Patient, Clarence Ward, 59
Pamment, James	Patient, 17, 23, 42, 63
Pamment, Liz	Mother of James, 17, 23, 63
Parkyn, Roy	Friend of Salina Townsend, 122, 140
Parsons, Sarah	Patient, Churchill Ward, 75, 77, 80
Patterson, Molly	Patient, Parrot Ward, 126

Q

Quinn, Stephen   Patient, Alice Ward, 38, 39

R

S

T

U

V

W